In this timely volume, Roger Frie and Pascal Sauvayre have gathered together a series of fascinating essays that take us back to a time when psychoanalysts engaged productively with the social sciences and the social world of their patients. The pioneering explorations of race, sexuality, and human relatedness chronicled here—many of them suppressed and forgotten—offer vivid testimony to the capaciousness and the radical possibilities of the interpersonal perspective in the clinical tradition. Full of unexpected pleasures, this book is a must-read for anyone concerned with the fate of psychoanalysis in our fractured world.

Elizabeth Lunbeck,
Professor of History of Science, Harvard University

The authors of this text have made a tremendous contribution to contemporary psychoanalysis by reviving the early and forgotten contributions made by the Interpersonal School that speak critically to the conformist attitudes and values embedded within our current practice. It provides a critical link for conceptualizing our present racial, political, economic, and social {dis-ease} through a much-needed psychoanalytic lens. This book is well done and needs to be read by early career and senior analysts alike.

Kirkland C. Vaughans,
Derner School of Psychology, Adelphi University

Finally! An insightful, politically-astute book that demonstrates the importance of interdisciplinary dialogue for addressing past and present issues of race, class and gender. Contributors look back to the pathbreaking first issue of the journal *Psychiatry* and examine a range of subjects from assimilation and conformity to criminal justice reform and the contemporary peril of fascism. Frie and Sauvayre's book should be assigned throughout psychology programs—it is that important to our profession and our society.

Philip Cushman,
author of *Constructing the Self, Constructing America*

I0031586

Culture, Politics and Race in the Making of Interpersonal Psychoanalysis

Culture, Politics and Race in the Making of Interpersonal Psychoanalysis traces the emergence of Interpersonal Psychoanalysis and demonstrates how the radical, cross-disciplinary dialogues that form its foundation are relevant to present-day social and cultural challenges.

Psychoanalysts today are grappling with how to address a host of societal and political crises. In the 1930s, a similar set of crises led a group of progressive practitioners and scholars to engage in a radical, cross-disciplinary dialogue that became the foundation for interpersonal psychoanalysis. Pioneering psychoanalysts created a form of thought and practice that viewed human suffering through the wider lens of society and culture and provided a means to address the pervasive issues of racism, sexuality and politics in human experience. With contributions from leading psychoanalysts and scholars, and by making use of original sources, this book evidences the significance of this approach to understanding marginalisation today.

Written in an open and accessible fashion, *Culture, Politics and Race in the Making of Interpersonal Psychoanalysis* demonstrates the importance of the early interpersonal-cultural school for the present moment. This book will appeal to a broad audience in psychoanalysis and psychotherapy, the history of medicine, and social and cultural theory.

Roger Frie is Professor of Education, Simon Fraser University, Affiliate Professor of Psychiatry, University of British Columbia, Vancouver, and Faculty and Supervisor, William Alanson White Institute, New York. He is an award-winning author and has published many books on human interaction, historical responsibility and cultural memory.

Pascal Sauvayre is faculty, supervising and training psychoanalyst at the William Alanson White Institute, New York. He studies and writes at the disciplinary boundaries of psychoanalysis, and he has a private practice in New York City.

Psychoanalysis in a New Key Book Series
Series Editor: Donnel Stern

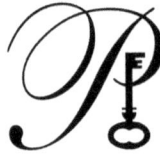

When music is played in a new key, the melody does not change, but the notes that make up the composition do: change in the context of continuity, continuity that perseveres through change. Psychoanalysis in a New Key publishes books that share the aims psychoanalysts have always had, but that approach them differently. The books in the series are not expected to advance any particular theoretical agenda, although to this date most have been written by analysts from the Interpersonal and Relational orientations.

The most important contribution of a psychoanalytic book is the communication of something that nudges the reader's grasp of clinical theory and practice in an unexpected direction. Psychoanalysis in a New Key creates a deliberate focus on innovative and unsettling clinical thinking. Because that kind of thinking is encouraged by exploration of the sometimes surprising contributions to psychoanalysis of ideas and findings from other fields, Psychoanalysis in a New Key particularly encourages interdisciplinary studies. Books in the series have married psychoanalysis with dissociation, trauma theory, sociology, and criminology. The series is open to the consideration of studies examining the relationship between psychoanalysis and any other field—for instance, biology, literary and art criticism, philosophy, systems theory, anthropology, and political theory.

But innovation also takes place within the boundaries of psychoanalysis, and Psychoanalysis in a New Key therefore also presents work that reformulates thought and practice without leaving the precincts of the field. Books in the series focus, for example, on the significance of personal values in psychoanalytic practice, on the complex interrelationship between the analyst's clinical work and personal life, on the consequences for the clinical situation when patient and analyst are from different cultures, and on the need for psychoanalysts to accept the degree to which they knowingly satisfy their own wishes during treatment hours, often to the patient's detriment. A full list of all titles in this series is available at: https://www.routledge.com/Psychoanalysis-in-a-New-Key-Book-Series/book-series/LEAPNKBS

Culture, Politics and Race in the Making of Interpersonal Psychoanalysis

Breaking Boundaries

Edited by
Roger Frie and Pascal Sauvayre

Routledge
Taylor & Francis Group
LONDON AND NEW YORK

First published 2022
by Routledge
4 Park Square, Milton Park, Abingdon, Oxon OX14 4RN

and by Routledge
605 Third Avenue, New York, NY 10158

Routledge is an imprint of the Taylor & Francis Group, an informa business

British Library Cataloguing-in-Publication Data
A catalogue record for this book is available from the British Library

Library of Congress Cataloging-in-Publication Data
A catalog record has been requested for this book

ISBN: 978-1-032-21866-3 (hbk)
ISBN: 978-1-032-21867-0 (pbk)
ISBN: 978-1-003-27035-5 (ebk)

DOI: 10.4324/9781003270355

Typeset in Times New Roman
by KnowledgeWorks Global Ltd.

Contents

Preface

This project is the result of our shared passion for interdisciplinary thinking and practice that goes back several decades. It began with our discovery of a key part of the history of the interpersonal-cultural tradition of psychoanalysis that seemed to have been forgotten by succeeding generations. The William Alanson White Institute of Psychiatry, Psychoanalysis and Psychology in New York City is known in the profession for its "interpersonal" point of view. For many years, Dr. Miltiades Zaphiropoulos had an office on the first floor of the Institute on West 74th Street. One of the bookshelves in his office contained multiple sets of professional journals. Amongst these was a journal whose early volumes reached back to 1938 and was distinguished by a distinct banner and the name *Psychiatry: The Journal of the Biology and the Pathology of Interpersonal Relations*.

The fact that the journal was in the possession of "Milt" or "Zaph," as he was known to his colleagues and students, was hardly fortuitous. Milt was the elder statesman of the Institute. He graduated in 1951 and passed away in 2015 at the age of 101. For many years, he was known as one of the Institute's unofficial historians. Milt's memory was prodigious and his own life seemed to mirror the many changes experienced by the psychoanalytic profession over the course of the twentieth century. Born into the ancient Greek community of Alexandria, Egypt, where his father was the harbor master, Milt attended university in Paris at the Sorbonne. He eventually found his way to the United States and was in the Navy during the Second World War. After the war, Milt became a member of one of the earliest cohorts of psychoanalytic trainees at the Institute. He seemed to have an exhaustive knowledge of psychoanalysis and was always available to answer questions. In one of our conversations, Milt recalled that when he was a young medical student in Paris in the 1930s, he had the pleasure of meeting Jacques Lacan. He had many such stories to tell, personal anecdotes that brought the history of the profession to life. That we should find a set of the journal, *Psychiatry*, in his office was somehow fitting.

The journal itself appeared pristine, which suggested it remained unopened over many years, possibly even decades. On the inside of the front cover was stamped, "Property of Ralph Crawley," one of the contributors to the first issue whose article is discussed in this volume. With its distinct banner and font in the modernist, international style of the 1930s, and with a special yellow-colored paper carefully chosen by the editorial board to enhance attention in the reader, the journal was more than simply a scholarly undertaking. It was an attempt to break with the norms of the time and directly challenge mainstream psychoanalytic scholarship. In short, *Psychiatry* stood out from the crowd from the very beginning, both in its material format and in its scholarly content.

As we leafed through the yellow, and perhaps just slightly "yellowed" pages from 1938, we imagined ourselves as intellectual archeologists. It is often said that history is there to be discovered and known. But the process of engaging the past is rarely straightforward. It requires us to recognize the limits of what we can know and to listen for voices that have been silenced or remain unheard. Freud once observed that it is only when the buried past is unearthed through the work of archeology that it begins to fade and disintegrate. Over time, Freud's observation became quite real for us as Crowley's pristine volume started to fall apart. We needed to learn how to work through its contents while preserving the journal for the present and future. This became an apt metaphor for the project as a whole. By analyzing the journal's texts, our project sought to break down and interpret their meanings in order to reconstruct and disclose new meaning – very much like the psychoanalytic process. The understanding we gained essentially spoke *from* the past *to* the present and future.

The first step was to choose the articles to be studied and to invite contributors. The authors of this volume were selected by the happenstance of our own interests and our connections in psychoanalysis and academia. As such, they represent not only our specific historical context but also our professional perspectives. Like us, most of the contributors are graduates of, or connected with, the William Alanson White Institute and we offered them articles to examine and write about. In all, approximately one-third of the articles published in Volume 1 of *Psychiatry* are explored and discussed here. Each reading proceeds differently: some contributors closely follow a text in order to challenge existing beliefs or capture voices that speak to the dynamics of gender, sexuality and race; other contributors use a text as a springboard for exploration and discussion of contemporary culture, society or politics.

While successive generations of clinicians may have overlooked the radicality of the early volumes of *Psychiatry*, the wider world of scholarship has been less neglectful. In 2011, for example, the historian of gender, sexuality and medicine, Naoko Wake, wrote an important intellectual biography, *Private practices: Harry Stack Sullivan, the science of homosexuality, and American liberalism*, that brought the interdisciplinary roots of the interpersonal-cultural school to light. Pascal reviewed that book for *Psychoanalytic Perspectives* and interviewed Prof. Wake as a complement to that review. A short time later, Roger wrote a detailed article in *Contemporary Psychoanalysis*, entitled "What is Cultural Psychoanalysis: Psychoanalytic Anthropology and Interpersonal Tradition," that examined the pathbreaking interdisciplinary work of the early interpersonal tradition. These publications substantiated our belief in the need for a broader study that would demonstrate the richness of cross-disciplinary dialogue and scholarship of the 1930s. This project is particularly important, we believe, at a time when we face social and political crises that would have been familiar to the authors who were published in Volume 1 of *Psychiatry*, and who themselves responded to the crises of the world around them through their actions and writing. We hope that this archeological project of "reaching back" into the radical interdisciplinary past can provide a more encompassing understanding of the present and a means to "reach forward" into the future.

Contributors

Julian Adler, J.D., is the director of policy and research at the Center for Court Innovation, a nonprofit that works to create a more effective and humane justice system by performing original research and helping launch reforms around the world. He leads the Center's work on a range of national initiatives, including the MacArthur Foundation's Safety and Justice Challenge. He is the co-author of *Start Here: A Road Map to Reducing Mass Incarceration* (The New Press), named one of the best books of 2018 by the Vera Institute of Justice and short-listed for the 2019 Media for a Just Society Award and for the Goddard Riverside Stephan Russo Book Prize for Social Justice. A licensed clinical social worker and an attorney, he was previously the director of the Red Hook Community Justice Center in Brooklyn, New York and led the planning process for Brooklyn Justice Initiatives.

Olivia Dana, J.D., is the deputy director of research-practice strategies at the Center for Court Innovation, where she works to improve justice system responses to both defendants and victims and to promote racial justice. She previously served as the director of the Staten Island Justice Center, which provides pretrial supervision, alternatives to incarceration and other community-based programming. Olivia began her career as a prosecutor in Brooklyn, New York. She holds a J.D. from the University of Michigan Law School.

Ann D'Ercole, Ph.D. ABPP., is a Clinical Associate Professor of Psychology at the New York University Postdoctoral Program in Psychotherapy and Psychoanalysis, where she is both teaching faculty and Supervisor. She is also Distinguished Visiting Faculty at the William Alanson White Institute and recipient of the APA, Division 39, Sexualities and Gender Identities Award for Outstanding Contributions to the Advancement of Sexualities and Gender Identities in Psychoanalysis. Her book, *Clara Thompson: The Life and Work of an American Psychoanalyst*, Routledge Press, is forthcoming. Dr. D'Ercole is in private practice in New York City.

Roger Frie is Professor of Education at Simon Fraser University and Affiliate Professor of Psychiatry at the University of British Columbia, both in Vancouver. He is also a graduate, supervisor and faculty member of the William Alanson White Institute and an Associate Member of the Columbia University Seminar on Cultural Memory in New York. He is an academic historian and philosopher and a psychoanalyst and psychologist in private practice. He writes and presents widely on the themes of historical responsibility, cultural memory and human interaction. He has published numerous interdisciplinary books and articles. He is author most recently of the award-winning book *Not in My Family: German Memory and Responsibility After the Holocaust* (Oxford University Press) and editor most recently of *History Flows Through Us: Germany, the Holocaust and the Importance of Empathy* (Routledge). He is editorial board member of *Contemporary Psychoanalysis*, *Psychoanalytic Discourse* and *Psychoanalytic Psychology* and a former editor of *Psychoanalysis, Self and Context*.

Orsolya Hunyady, Ph.D., is a clinical psychologist, psychoanalyst, practising in New York City. She teaches and supervises in several training programs at the William Alanson White Institute, and is an Assistant Editor for *Contemporary Psychoanalysis*. She has been publishing articles and book chapters on psychoanalytic subjects with an emphasis on their cultural, social and historical context.

Victoria Malkin, Ph.D., LP., has a Ph.D. in anthropology from University College, London, and is a psychoanalyst in private practice in New York City. She teaches as an adjunct professor at the New School for Social Research. She has published articles on the area of gender, migration and identity. She is on the Editorial Boards of *The Psychoanalytic Review* and *Contemporary Psychoanalysis.*

Katharina Rothe, Ph.D., is a clinical psychologist, psychoanalyst and psychosocial researcher. She is a graduate of psychoanalytic training at the William Alanson White Institute in New York where she also teaches the course *Gender, Sex & Sexuality.* Alongside maintaining a private practice in New York City, she is widely published in academic journals and books on psychoanalysis, qualitative methods in psychoanalytic social research, sex and gender, anti-Semitism, racism, the aftermath of National Socialism and the Holocaust. She is an editor of the German journal *Psychoanalyse. Texte zur Sozialforschung* [Psychoanalysis, Contributions to Social Research] and on the editorial board of *Contemporary Psychoanalysis.* In 2021, her translation of a major essay by Alfred Lorenzer will be published by UIT as a book entitled "Cultural Analysis Now!"

Pascal Sauvayre, Ph.D., is faculty, supervising analyst and training analyst at the William Alanson White Institute. He writes and publishes at the interdisciplinary borders of psychoanalysis. His recent projects include contributing and editing *The Unconscious: Contemporary Refractions in Psychoanalysis* (2020: Routledge), and projects in press include contributing to *Renewing Hermeneutics: Thinking with Paul Ricoeur* (2021: Inschibboleth), editing the English translation of Tomàs Casado's and María Herrero's *Early Relational Trauma and the Development of the Self* (2022: Routledge), contributing to the volume translating Alfred Lorenzer's "In-Depth Hermeneutical Cultural Analysis" (est. 2021: The Unconscious in Translation), and translating Jean Laplanche's *The Analyst's Tub: Transcendence of the Transference* (est. 2021: The Unconscious in Translation). He has a private practice in New York City.

Michelle Stephens is Dean of the Humanities and Professor of English and Latino and Caribbean Studies at Rutgers University, New Brunswick. She is also a graduate, supervisor and faculty member of the William Alanson White Institute and a practising psychoanalyst. She writes on black literary and performance studies, Caribbean art and visuality, and the emerging field of Archipelagic American Studies. Among other works, she is the author of *Black Empire: The Masculine Global Imaginary of Caribbean Intellectuals in the United States, 1914 to 1962* (Duke University Press, 2005), *Skin Acts: Race, Psychoanalysis and The Black Male Performer* (Duke, 2014), *Archipelagic American Studies*, co-edited with Brian Russell Roberts (Duke, 2017) and the exhibition catalog *Relational Undercurrents: Contemporary Art of the Caribbean Archipelago*, co-edited with Tatiana Flores (Duke, 2017).

Naoko Wake is Associate Professor of History and the Director of the Asian Pacific American Studies Program at Michigan State University. A historian of gender, sexuality and illness in the Pacific region, she has authored *Private Practices: Harry Stack Sullivan, the Science of Homosexuality, and American Liberalism* (Rutgers, 2011) on the history of psychiatric and psychoanalytic approaches to homosexuality, and *American Survivors: Trans-Pacific Memories of Hiroshima and Nagasaki* (Cambridge, 2021), which explores the history of Asian American survivors of 1945 atomic bombings. Her current project is the history of disability in Asian Pacific Islander Desi American families and communities.

Figures

The Sociocultural Turn

An Introduction

Roger Frie and Pascal Sauvayre

At a time when society is becoming ever more compartmentalized, riven by political, economic and racial divisions, binary thinking can hold a strong appeal. The need to create avenues of interaction that challenge entrenched differences has rarely been greater. But attempts to break through established boundaries can stir controversy. As a profession, psychoanalysis is no stranger to controversy. By encouraging a diversity of ideas and actions, radical forms of psychoanalysis have long opposed binary modes of thinking.

In the 1930s, the interpersonal-cultural tradition of psychoanalysis emerged out a groundbreaking cross-disciplinary dialogue that involved the psychological professions, social scientists, the humanities and the sciences writ large. The practitioners and scholars involved in this dialogue believed in the need to confront and change existing societal inequities even as they were themselves affected and shaped by the social and political forces of the period. Western societies at the time were undergoing a period of deep turmoil. The decade of 1930s was characterized by a host of social and geopolitical crises. The United States was in the grip of the Great Depression and the American South was ruled by Jim Crow. Racial and societal inequities were widespread. In Europe, the rise of fascist governments in Germany and Italy threatened the stability of democratic regimes. By the end of the decade, the aggressive territorial expansions of Nazi Germany in Europe and Imperial Japan in south-east Asia plunged the world into a long and vicious global war. In the years that followed, Nazi Germany's perpetration of the Holocaust and Imperial Japan's war crimes against Asian-Pacific nations shed

DOI: 10.4324/9781003270355-1

light on the depth of human destructiveness and the need for a charter of human rights.

This geopolitical foment affected the development of psychoanalysis in a number of ways, the most visible of which was the emigration of many of its luminaries to locations outside of continental Europe. In the United States, a transplanted strand of psychoanalytic practice and thinking was established. European psychoanalytic émigrés, many of whom were Jewish, began to work with American colleagues, and injected a new energy into burgeoning schools of analytic thought even as they sought to manage their own traumatic losses.

In the 1930s, the problem of human sociality took on an importance that went well beyond the clinical setting or the academy. Questions about how people interacted with one another, the way in which human well-being is linked to others, and the role that society, culture, politics and race play in this process, became more pressing. The attempt to answer these and other similar questions spurred an intellectual milieu that not only welcomed but actively fostered interdisciplinary dialogue and debate. The aim of this book is to show just how radical this period of learning and intellectual exchange really was. Not only did it lay the foundation for the interpersonal-cultural perspective that we know today as interpersonal psychoanalysis, it helped create a form of thought and practice that viewed human suffering through a wider lens of social and cultural forces, norms and values. Indeed, the linking of the individual to culture and society is what set this new "interpersonal" perspective apart from the profession of psychoanalysis as a whole.

We face many social and political crises today that would likely have been familiar to those who lived through the turmoil of the 1930s: a shift towards fascist forms of government, systemic forms discrimination and racial terror, an egregious wealth gap caused by destructive, unfettered capitalism, the cascading effects of a climate emergency and a global pandemic. Notwithstanding the historical specificity of our current situation, the parallels to the 1930s require us to ask what we can learn from the past, and to consider how we might apply those insights to the present and future.

Psychoanalysis today is often seen as an embattled profession. Many within the psychoanalytic community have sought closer links with the medical sciences and the neurosciences in particular. While this approach has many merits, we believe that the need to think about and engage ways of thinking and practicing from disciplines in the social sciences and humanities is equally, if not more, compelling and urgent. We suggest that a return to the kind of groundbreaking cross-disciplinary work of the 1930s can be instructive and shed light on the continued necessity for more, not less, interdisciplinarity in the profession.

There is also another important factor at work. The current social and political crises have led many psychoanalysts from all schools, but perhaps especially from the interpersonal, relational and Lacanian varieties, to speak directly to the deleterious effects of negative social forces such as racism, vast economic disparities, authoritarianism and fanaticism. Thus, it seems an auspicious moment in which to return to the radicality of an earlier period and to ask not only what we can learn, but also, perhaps, what happened to that radical spark? How might conformist impulses within these movements have blunted their efficacy? For example, in the latter half of the twentieth century, as interpersonal psychoanalysis became more established, it also became ever more professionalized and distant from its origins. How do we ensure that the current rise in progressive thinking within psychoanalysis is not lost yet again?

Radical Interdisciplinary Roots

The roots of the interpersonal perspective can be traced back to the establishment in 1938 of the journal *Psychiatry: Journal of the Biology and Pathology of Interpersonal Relations*. The founding editor, Harry Stack Sullivan, was insistent that the name of the new journal not include the term "psychoanalysis." The stated goal was to explore the spaces between psychiatry, psychoanalysis, the social sciences and the humanities, in essence to learn from their interaction. Indeed, although named *Psychiatry*, the journal's mission statement makes clear that it is intended for "all serious students of human living in any of its aspects" (William Alanson White Psychiatric Foundation, 1938, p. ii). The four issues that make up Volume 1 of *Psychiatry* embody Sullivan's cross-disciplinary ambitions. They include contributions from fields as diverse as sociology, anthropology, philosophy, political science, law, economics, business, biology, psychiatry and psychoanalysis. The

writers themselves were giants in their fields and include such luminaries as the anthropologists Ruth Benedict and Edward Sapir and
the political scientist Harold Laswell to name but a few.

The journal's first editorial (Sullivan, 1938) highlights the fact that it
is guided by an interdisciplinary "nucleus" (p. 137) of four experts: a
psychiatrist (Sullivan), a political scientist (Laswell), an anthropologist
(Sapir) and a psychoanalyst (Ernest Hadley). The objective is to embrace
"research into almost any aspect of people and interpersonal relations, broadly conceived" (p. 141). Particularly noteworthy, especially
in light of our contemporary situation, is that "political discontent" is
announced as a central concern of the journal, which will be studied
by means of "political psychiatry" (pp. 136–137). The different disciplinary viewpoints were all linked by a common objective: to demonstrate the relevance of diverse ideas and thus to educate, challenge and
enlarge the worldview of the practicing clinician and interested reader.
The inaugural issues of *Psychiatry* stood out as a significant departure from prevailing psychoanalytic scholarship at the time, and their
contents continue to stand out today. Indeed, it is hard to think of any
contemporary psychoanalytic journal that so actively fosters the kind
of broad cross-disciplinary aims embodied by *Psychiatry* in 1938.

We believe there is much to be learned from looking more closely at
this formative example of early interdisciplinary research and scholarship. Our aim in putting together this edited volume is to create a
dialogue that links the past and the present, one that draws on the creative impulse of the early interpersonal-cultural perspective to meet
the challenges facing us today. Above all, we believe that this unique
history needs to be more widely known. The kind of historical understanding we have in mind has a fundamentally important educative
objective. In the most basic sense, knowledge of history can help us to
respond to the present without repeating the mistakes of the past. But
beyond this, the radical cross-disciplinary nature of early interpersonal scholarship challenged binary thinking at the time and is especially relevant today as society is increasingly threatened by similar
kinds of reductionist thought and action.

The open and inclusive outlook of the early interpersonalists stood
in stark contrast to the mainstream psychoanalytic thinking of the
time, especially in North America. From 1937 onwards, mainstream
psychoanalysis explicitly identified as a member of the medical

sciences by limiting training to psychiatrists and eschewed its human-istic, interdisciplinary roots. This resulted in a protracted insularity that contributed to the rejection and banishment of interpersonalism, with its embrace of a plurality of voices, for many decades.

While early interpersonalists engaged in questions pertaining to society and politics and found ways to respond to the rapidly deterio-rating events of the time, mainstream psychoanalysts tended to avoid the social and political altogether, believing them to be less relevant to the internal workings of the mind. In the face of today's societal and political crises, the profession of psychoanalysis cannot afford to repeat the same kind of mistakes. Over time, however, as the interpersonal-cultural perspective became more established, we believe it also defaulted to a kind of insularity that led to a neglect of its own progressive origins. We maintain that the courage and creative-ness of the authors who published their work in the inaugural issues of *Psychiatry* stand as a testament and example for how we should attend to our own professional, political and cultural surround today.

At the end of *Psychiatry's* first decade, Sullivan (1947, pp. 433–435) reviewed 350 items that had appeared in its pages. Sullivan reported that apart from mental health professionals, the 197 authors whose work was published in the journal included 19 sociologists, 13 anthro-pologists, 7 political scientists, 6 educators, 4 social workers, 3 lawyers, 2 philosophers and 2 historians. As these findings suggest, the journal remained true to its interdisciplinary origins throughout the first dec-ade of its publication. Yet these statistics tell only part of the story. The diversity of the authors should also be considered. At the time, white, heterosexual, Christian males made up the majority of the psy-chological sciences and academic professions. It is noteworthy, there-fore, that in the first volume of *Psychiatry* alone, African-American, Asian American, gay, lesbian, Jewish and female authors were all rep-resented. This suggests that the radicality of the journal lay not just in its interdisciplinarity, but in the fact that many of the contributors spoke as outsiders – as others – in a society where power and privilege lay in the hands of straight white men.

The stories of the authors, and the issue of marginalization they speak to and embody, are a touchstone of this volume. At a time in which psychoanalysts are again seeking to address the deep lack of diversity in their profession, revealing this hidden history strikes us as particularly important. Of course, as progressive as the upstart journal, its editors and authors may have been, they were still ensconced in the majority white culture of the time. Even as they sought to challenge cultural meaning and norms, many of the authors seemed unaware of the degree to which they remained embedded in a conservative societal outlook. Thus, we find contradictions and tensions: an exclusively white, male editorial board that published a diversity of voices, seemingly without recognizing its own privilege, or authors who took up controversial subjects of the time, only to end supporting normative social values and the status quo. This points to the degree to which we always struggle to be aware of our own embeddedness in sociocultural contexts that inevitably shape our perspective on the world.

The first decade of *Psychiatry* was also relevant in other ways. This period saw the push towards establishing educational institutions that would enable an interdisciplinary and radical impulse to find fruition for a new generation of practicing clinicians. In 1936, the Washington School of Psychiatry was founded and embodied Sullivan's belief in the need for a cross-disciplinary medical education of psychiatrists. The 1930s were a time when psychoanalytically oriented psychiatrists and those interested in the question of "life-history" were open to working with a range of psychoanalysts from different professional backgrounds. This process of cross-disciplinary learning and practice reached its height in 1943, when Harry Stack Sullivan, Erich Fromm, Frieda Fromm-Reichman and Clara Thompson joined together with David Rioch, a research neurophysiologist, and Janet Rioch, a pediatrician, to establish the William Alanson White Institute of Psychiatry, Psychoanalysis and Psychology in New York. The institute was named in honor of William Alanson White, who died in 1937. White was a leading early twentieth century American psychiatrist whose views on clinical practice at the time had an influence on many of his students, perhaps most notably on Sullivan himself.[1]

The importance of William Alanson White for the emergence of interpersonal psychoanalysis, and for psychoanalytic psychiatry more generally, cannot be underestimated (see D'Amore, 1976). White was a prolific author, progressive in his views on criminal reform and care of the mentally ill. As an early opponent of capital punishment, he argued for the importance of understanding how individuals are shaped by their interactions and social contexts (White, 1933).[2] As White (1928, p. 128) states, "I am thinking, for instance, of the study of the individual, not solely as an individual, but in his dynamic relations with his fellows." Over the course of his career, White was president of the American Psychiatric Association and American Psychoanalytic Association and played an important role in the dissemination of psychoanalytic knowledge and practice. In 1913, he co-founded the *Psychoanalytic Review*, the first English language psychoanalytic journal, and asserted the need to broaden medical and psychoanalytic education through the inclusion of other disciplines, especially the social sciences. As the superintendent of Saint Elizabeth's Hospital in Washington, DC, White was a mentor and friend to Harry Stack Sullivan. Together, they shared in the belief that a full accounting of the person was dependent on understanding what the social sciences could teach us.

The interdisciplinary perspectives of White and Sullivan would find fruition in the new training programs established in Washington and New York. For White, the Berlin Institute formed an important educative model, so it was perhaps not surprising that Fromm, a graduate of the Berlin Institute, and a faculty member of the Washington School of Psychiatry and William Alanson White Institute, would assert that "Psychology cannot be divorced from philosophy and ethics nor from sociology and economics" (Fromm, 1947, p. ix). Sadly, the optimism that imbued this new educative approach was not widely shared. The history of the field suggests that psychoanalytic institutes have generally resisted establishing an interdisciplinary approach to training. We believe this has much to do with the nature of clinical education in the psychological professions which, over time, became ever more focused on clinical and technical detail. Clinical endeavors, moreover, were increasingly distinguished from the study of human experience in other disciplines, with the result that the extensive interconnections between them have often gone unnoted. In contrast, and in line with White, Sullivan, Fromm and others, we believe strongly in the need for psychoanalysts to engage in cross-disciplinary thinking and practice and thus to create opportunities for the kind of radical learning that was once available but lost as a result of institutional and disciplinary boundary setting.

Emergence of Interpersonal Psychoanalysis

The term "interpersonal psychoanalysis" is today an accepted part of psychoanalytic and professional lexicon. It is important, therefore, to underline that in 1938, when *Psychiatry* was first published, the term had not yet come into existence. Sullivan explicitly resisted describing his approach as "psychoanalysis," preferring "psychiatry" instead. It was not until 1964 that Maurice Green, a graduate of the William Alanson White Institute, coined the term "interpersonal psychoanalysis" in his edited book, *Interpersonal psychoanalysis: The selected papers of Clara Thompson*. In the preface to that work, Green writes that "Thompson's emphasis, in theory as well as in practice, was always concentrating on and analyzing what went on between persons to facilitate the growth of a human relationship – what I would call 'interpersonal psychoanalysis'" (Green, 1964, p. vi). Even if the term "interpersonal psychoanalysis" was used before 1964, it was neither a common nor official designation and its evolution points to the intersection of different disciplines and viewpoints.

Sullivan may have identified first and foremost as a psychiatrist, but Fromm, Fromm-Reichmann and Thompson were all psychoanalysts. Fromm and Fromm-Reichmann had a history of psychoanalytic engagement in Germany. Fromm-Reichmann was a psychiatrist, and after training at the Berlin Institute of Psychoanalysis, she founded a psychoanalytic sanatorium in 1924. Fromm was a sociologist and entered into an analysis with Fromm-Reichmann, which ended after they fell in love. They were married in 1926 and became co-founders, with Karl Landauer, of the Southwest German Psychoanalytic Institute in Frankfurt in 1927. Fromm underwent a further analysis with Wilhelm Wittenberg in Munich and subsequently moved to Berlin in 1928 to finish his psychoanalytic training at the Institute there and complete his training analysis with Hanns Sachs, an early disciple of Freud.

Like Fromm-Reichmann, Thompson was a psychiatrist with a strong interest in psychoanalysis. After reading Ferenczi's work and attending a lecture he gave during a visit to New York, Thompson asked if he would become her analyst. Ferenczi encouraged Thompson to come to Budapest for treatment. She travelled to Budapest for three summers and in 1931 moved there to finish her analysis. Thompson returned to New York in 1934, joining Sullivan who already lived in the city. For a short period of time, Thompson even became Sullivan's analyst. Fromm also arrived in the city in 1934, followed by Frieda Fromm-Reichmann in 1935. In the years that followed, Sullivan, Thompson, Fromm and Fromm-Reichmann, together with Karen Horney, worked to account for the primacy of social and cultural factors in human development. As a group, they traced the etiology of neuroses to social and cultural experience, rather than biology, which distinguished them from Freud and the psychoanalytic mainstream. There were of course many individual differences between them, and Horney would go her separate way by 1943. But they were all linked by a shared commitment to move beyond Freud's biological emphasis and develop a social and culture account of human experience.

While Sullivan can justifiably be recognized as establishing a path for other interpersonal psychoanalysts to follow, during the decades of the 1940s and 1950s, the foundation for the term "interpersonal psychoanalysis" was laid first by Fromm and then Thompson. Perhaps the earliest and clearest indication of this new direction can be found in the Appendix of Fromm's 1941 bestseller, *Escape from Freedom*. Fromm explains the role of society and culture in the shaping of the individual and then goes on to declare that:

> In our opinion, the fundamental approach to human personality is the understanding of the human being's relationship to the world, to others, to nature, and to him or herself. We believe that the human being is *primarily* a social being, and not, as Freud assumes, primarily self-sufficient and only secondarily in need of others in order to satisfy his or her instinctual needs. In this sense, we believe that individual psychology is fundamentally social psychology, or in Sullivan's terms, the psychology of interpersonal relationships; the key problem of psychology is that of the particular kind of relatedness of the individual towards the world, not that of satisfaction or frustration of single instinctual desires. The problem of what happens to the person's instinctual desires has to be understood as one part of the total problem of his or her relationship towards the world and not as *the* problem of human personality. Therefore, in our approach, the needs and

desires that center about the individual's relations to others, such
as love, hatred, tenderness, symbiosis, are the fundamental psychological phenomena.

(Fromm, 1941, p. 290)

In 1947, shortly after the end of World War II and the founding of
the Institute, Fromm explicitly ties the psychology of interpersonal
relationships to psychoanalysis, writing in his *Man for himself* that:

The progress of psychoanalytic theory led, in line with the progress of the natural and social sciences, to a new concept which
was based, not on the idea of a primarily isolated individual, but on
the *relationship* of man to others, to nature, and to him or herself...
H. S. Sullivan, one of the pioneers of this new view, has accordingly
defined psychoanalysis as a "study of interpersonal relations.

(1947, p. 57)

By 1949, when Sullivan suddenly died, he had already become less
involved in the running of the new institute in New York. In 1950,
Fromm moved to Mexico, though he continued to spend many months
each year teaching and supervising at the institute. Over the following decade, Thompson develops the interpersonal perspective, be it
through the running of the institute (she was the first Director) or the
manner in which she wove together aspects of Sullivan's interpersonal
theory with Ferenczi's and Fromm's psychoanalytic perspectives to
create a new whole. For example, in her 1955 address, *The history of
the William Alanson White Institute*, Thompson uses the term "interpersonal theory" (see D'Ercole, in press). In a paper on the work of
Ferenczi, she uses the term "interpersonal relations" (1988, p. 194).
And in her discussion of Sullivan and psychoanalysis, she employs the
terms "interpersonal process" (1978, p. 496), "interpersonal forces"
(1978, p. 50) and "interpersonal relations" (1978, p. 492). In other
words, when Green coined "interpersonal psychoanalysis," he was
capturing the work and spirit of an emergent tradition. Given the intersection of ideas up to that point, it is not surprising to find that Fromm
wrote the Forward to the volume of Thompson's selected papers. An
oft overlooked fact is that Fromm was also Thompson's third analyst,
thus completing what might best be described as "a circle of influence"
between the main founders of interpersonal psychoanalysis.

The Cultural School of Psychoanalysis

We both began our psychoanalytic training at the William Alanson White Institute in the early to mid-1990s. At the time, we would occasionally hear mention of a so-called cultural school of psychoanalysis. Yet everything about the term seemed to be shrouded in mystery. Upon inquiring further, we learned that from the late 1930s, the term "cultural psychoanalysis" was the accepted designation of the emerging interpersonal tradition. The fact that the cultural school name was, and has, remained relatively little known among our Institute colleagues, let alone in the wider psychoanalytic profession, points to the central, and often problematic question of culture that this volume will address (see Frie, 2014).

In fact, this seemingly benign term had become hostage to the psychoanalytic politics of the era, in particular the thorny relationship between the early interpersonalists and their "orthodox" Freudian colleagues. Over the decades, even some interpersonalists experienced the label, ecome hostage to the psychoanalytic politics of the era, in particular the thorny relationship between the early interpersonalists interpersonal tradition as a form of social relativism and conformism. After all, if psychological experience was entirely determined by social and cultural forces, what place was left for the individual psyche? The fact that Fromm had expressly argued against social relativism and adaptation in *Escape from Freedom* seemed to make little impact on the critics: "In trying to avoid the errors of biological and metaphysical concepts we must not succumb to an equally grave error, that of a sociological relativism in which the person is nothing but a puppet, directed by the strings of social circumstances" (Fromm, 1941, p. 289). The mainstream psychoanalytic establishment would have none of it.

We may appreciate the consternation that early generations of interpersonalists must have felt about the cultural school label, given that their place in the psychoanalytic professional world was hardly secure. The desire for acceptance and recognition was strong. Since that time, however, the evolution of psychoanalytic thinking and practice has grown to embrace a broad sociocultural turn, making the situation appear different today. From our contemporary vantage point, we think it is fair to say that the cultural school label demonstrates the forward-looking nature of the early interpersonalists, who sought to bridge culture, society and psychoanalysis. Culture, in the broad sense it was used at the time, could refer both to the culture of ethnic groups and to the social systems that shape human interaction and the interpretation of meaning.

Of course, the question that must be asked, is what happened to the attempt to bridge the study of culture and psychoanalysis? By mid-century, the drive to maintain an interdisciplinary dialogue between psychoanalysis and related disciplines like anthropology or sociology, which were prominently represented in the early volumes of *Psychiatry*, had dissipated. For many psychoanalysts, regardless of orientation, the period of "excursions into interdisciplinary theorizing" increasingly posed a threat to "an analytic community that was anxious to protect the autonomy of psychoanalysis as a scientific discipline" (Manson, 1988, p. 112). The roots of this reaction can be traced back to Freud who, with some of the same anxieties, would approach other disciplines as "interdisciplinary contests" (Winter, 1999) that needed to be won.

The preoccupation with establishing psychoanalysis as a medical science meant that questions of culture, society and politics were increasingly ignored. For the majority of mainstream psychoanalytic practitioners, the disciplines of anthropology and sociology could do little to advance a properly scientific account of the analytic relationship. The singular focus on the patient's intrapsychic experience meant that sociocultural contexts were seen separate, or subordinate to and derivative of the intra-psychic realm. In addition, there was another important factor at work. Those psychoanalysts who continued to maintain an active interest in the study of society and culture became increasingly identified with the growing revisionist perspective that challenged mainstream Freudian theory and practice. Thus, to the extent they were recognized at all, they came to occupy a place on the periphery of the psychoanalytic profession, above all in independent institutes that existed outside of the mainstream American Psychoanalytic Association or the International Psychoanalytic Association.

But here another question emerges. Since the William Alanson White Institute was not part of the mainstream, and presumably was not under the same organizational pressures, what happened to the early sociocultural impulse we discuss in this book? Were the radical interdisciplinary perspectives of the 1930s simply lost over time, as the professionalization of psychoanalysis began to dominate? Or was the explicit focus on the interpersonal, therapeutic dyad in fact undertaken at the cost of understanding and examining the generative influence of social and political forces on the individual *and* the relationship? And how might the radical spark of the 1930s intersect with contemporary concerns about social and political forces?

In today's sociocultural perspective, certainly, psychological life is seen as shaped by social, cultural and political forces that often exist outside of our awareness. As psychological beings, we are not merely facilitated, but actually constituted by these forces. We are born into cultural contexts that provide us with the tools and means to understand and express ourselves (see Frie, 2011, 2013, 2014). We are participants in the process of culture. How we think about ourselves or others is always and inevitably limited by and representative of the cultural values and norms in which we exist. This applies as much to individuals as it does to the theories we hold dear and that we too often believe to be universal in nature. Yet because each of us possess a unique history and particular perspective within culture, we also have the potential to effect the context in which we exist. As editors of this volume, we believe it is important to view culture not as a static entity that can be reified, but rather, as an inherently dynamic, participatory and interactive process that shapes the work we do and the goals we set out in therapeutic practice. The viewpoint we are describing takes as its starting point our unconscious embeddedness in a world of social and cultural interaction and rejects persisting dichotomies between the inner and outer, mind and context, I and other. Human experience always unfolds within the possibilities set forth by the shared meanings that our culture provides. Indeed, a major theme running throughout the chapters of this volume is to shed light on the meanings of culture.

Psychoanalysts, their patients and the psychoanalytic process itself are inalterably shaped by the language, values and norms of their culture and society. This perspective has important ramifications. When culture is reduced to a single ethnic group, or when understandings of culture are limited to talk of diversity and difference, then we overlook the degree to which *all* persons are inescapably embedded in culture. The fact is that members of the majority group in our society tend to think of themselves as cultureless. As a result, portrayals of culture belonging to the dominant group are often superficial, and systemic values and norms, as well as differences in language use, education, religious persuasion or economic background are neglected. Above all, the pervasiveness of racism as a structural problem, not just as an individual issue, is neglected, if not altogether denied. This volume seeks to contribute to the shift away from a reductionistic emphasis on the primacy of the "individual" in order to recognize the primacy of sociocultural contexts and systems, from which the meaning of the subject is constructed through interaction with others.

Plan of the Book

The contributors to this book are all linked by their interdisciplinary backgrounds and interests. In creating this volume, we asked contributors to draw on their expertise and reflect on one or more articles from the inaugural volume of *Psychiatry*. The aim of each chapter is twofold. First, to help readers appreciate the scope of the interdisciplinary perspectives represented by authors from the 1930s, and second, to reflect on the ways in which our own contemporary setting, especially as related to culture, politics and race, might benefit from a renewed cross-disciplinary approach that learns from the past and also speaks to the present. As we stated at the outset, we face a host of crises today. How might we use the generative impulse of a radical past to confront some of the myriad crises we face, be it as a profession or as a society? And what may we be overlooking as a result of ideas and beliefs that we hold dear or are hesitant to criticize? Beginning with a chapter on Sullivan, this volume explores seminal issues of culture, racism, feminism, sexuality and politics in the making of interpersonal psychoanalysis, and concludes with chapters on two other founders of interpersonal psychoanalysis, Thompson and Fromm.

We invited Naoko Wake, author of the pathbreaking intellectual biography of Harry Stack Sullivan (2011), to open our volume. Chapter 1, *The Roots of Interpersonal Psychoanalysis: Harry S. Sullivan, Interdisciplinary Inquiry, and Subjectivity* focuses on the radical cross-disciplinary dialogue of the 1930s that formed the basis for the emergence of interpersonal psychoanalysis. The chapter details the Culture and Personality seminar at Yale University that was organized by Edward Sapir and created a synergy between anthropologists, sociologists and psychoanalytic psychiatrists. The seminar offered Sullivan the opportunity to develop an interdisciplinary per-spective on life histories across contexts: sexual, social, political and racial. The seminar also provided a model for future educational institutes and for the advancement of psychoanalysis more generally. Indeed, as this chapter suggests, the need to understand, challenge and overcome traditional boundaries of thought and practice is an essential aspect of the interpersonal approach.

In Chapter 2, *Anthropology and Psychoanalysis: A Lost Dialogue Over Time*, Victoria Malkin explores the extent to which anthropol-ogy and psychoanalysis share a heritage in their conceptualizations of culture and the other. As Malkin shows, each field searched for a mas-ter narrative that could grasp human experience. But anthropology and psychoanalysis followed different paths, and this distance con-tinues to shape their lack of interaction today. Her chapter provides insight into why the two fields have been so misaligned. Drawing on two articles by Edward Sapir (1938) and Ruth Benedict (1938), Malkin examines the early history of dialogue between anthropology and psychoanalysis and asks what it would mean for psychoanalysis to take in anthropological thinking as something more than anecdotal data about a distant Other. She challenges narrow, outdated concep-tions of culture and asks whether an actual dialogue with anthropol-ogy might not put cherished psychoanalytic ideas at risk.

In Chapter 3, *More Simply Human Than Otherwise: Interpersonal Psychoanalysis and the Field of the "Negro Problem,"* Michelle Stephens examines Harry Stack Sullivan's important yet often overlooked fieldwork in the American southern and middle states during the late 1930s and early 1940s, along with his 1938 editorial on anti-Semitism. Together, this work (Sullivan, 1938, 1940, 1963) enables us to reflect on what Sullivan's approach has to offer the study of, and clinical practice within, the field of American race relations. As Stevens shows, in the late 1930s and early 1940s, the racial field included researchers across racial lines who studied interracial encounters and the interracial problem of "the Negro." The brevity of the moment, and the fleeting nature of the interactions between white psychosocial researchers and the subjects that black imaginative thinkers like Ralph Ellison and Richard Wright wrote about, represents a lost opportunity. But as Stevens demonstrates, it is an important achievement that is worth revisiting, especially with contemporary events in mind.

In Chapter 4, *Philosophical Foundations of Interpersonal Psychoanalysis: Alfred Dunham Jr. and Racial Politics*, Pascal Sauvayre examines the long-overlooked philosophical work of Alfred Dunham Jr. (1938), the only African-American author and scholar included in the first issue of *Psychiatry*. Sullivan's decision to foreground Dunham Jr.'s philosophical treatise on the concept of tension is important on multiple levels. In examining the work of Dunham Jr., we add to our understanding of the interdisciplinary role of philosophy for psychoanalysis. But it also raises a significant question about the place of African-American philosophy that has been generally if not entirely overlooked by psychoanalysis. Most importantly, this chapter considers the reasons why Dunham Jr.'s contribution, along with the work of other African-American writers and subjects outlined by Stevens in the previous chapter, have been neglected, even when Sullivan uses Dunham Jr.'s work to develop some of his most groundbreaking interpersonal concepts. The effects of racism in the intellectual trajectory of interpersonal psychoanalysis are considered, and the lost opportunities through the implicit and explicit dismissal of African-American philosophy are made evident.

In Chapter 5, *Reproduction and Resistance: Psychoanalysis in the Midst of the Political Economy*, Katharina Rothe explores the sociopolitical dimensions and struggles embedded in the evolution of psychoanalysis and "mental health" more generally. Rothe draws on Kingsley Davis's "Mental Hygiene and the Class Structure" (1938), and J. F. Brown's "Freud vs. Marx: Real and Pseudo Problems Distinguished" (1938) to rethink the interdisciplinary and political roots of psychoanalysis. Rothe examines the role and thought of Erich Fromm and the Frankfurt School of Social Research to consider how psychoanalytic schools have remained entrenched and boxed-in, even when their emphasis is to undo the binaries and boundaries that not only limit, but also destroy, human potential. Rothe suggests that the compartmentalization of disciplines reproduces the larger sociopolitical forces that these schools, and interpersonal psychoanalysis, so eloquently critique.

In Chapter 6, *Do Less Harm: Notes on Clinical Practice in the Age of Criminal Justice Reform*, Julian Adler and Olivia Dana suggest that far from self-executing and liberatory, the intersection of psychoanalysis and the law may be a site where normative boundaries are more easily reinforced than broken. They undertake a close reading of Ralph M. Crowley's "The Courts and Psychiatry" (1938) to underscore the risk that clinicians may lend further credence to biases enshrined in the criminal law (in Crowley's case, homophobia). Adler and Dana suggest that with the opening of the first drug court in Miami-Dade County, Florida in 1989, and the subsequent rise of specialized courts and diversion programs throughout the United States, an increasing number of clinicians are being hired to provide therapeutic interventions in criminal justice settings. By way of conclusion, the chapter points to a potential paradigm shift toward an ecological perspective that could serve to both mitigate this risk of bias and better align clinical practice with the project of humanizing the American justice system.

In Chapter 7, *Immigrants in Our Own Country: Responsibility Towards the Past and Future of Interpersonal Psychoanalysis*, Orsolya Hunyady explores the experience of Elizabeth Weigert-Vowinkel through her article "The Cult and Mythology of the Magna Mater from the Standpoint of Psychoanalysis" (1938). Weigert's discussion of gender and culture challenged traditional psychoanalysis and marked her own transition from being an early devotee of Freud in her native Germany, to being an émigré psychoanalyst in Turkey and then the United States. Hunyady suggests that the psychological dynamics of the forced immigration of European analysts, along with the conditions and values that dominated the United States at the time, led to the emergence of a combative and diverse psychoanalytic scene. But the valorization of assimilation and conformity in the 1930s meshed with an emphasis on self-sufficiency and individualism that pushed the political and economic system steadily rightward. The chapter concludes with an examination of the Hungarian émigré philosopher, Ágnes Heller, and suggests that if psychoanalysis wants to preserve its relevance and avoid being coopted, it needs to embrace its current marginal, subversive position.

In Chapter 8, *Considering the Radical Contributions of Clara Mabel Thompson*, Ann d'Ercole sheds light on Clara Thompson's pivotal role in the emergence of interpersonal psychoanalysis. D'Ercole undertakes a detailed reading of Thompson's "Notes on the Psychoanalytic Significance of the Choice of Analyst" (1938), to consider her radical contributions. The historical and geographical contexts of Thompson's life are considered and their influence on her values, lifestyle and way of thinking are demonstrated. Above all, d'Ercole shows the role played by Thompson's interaction with Sandor Ferenczi during the early 1930s and traces her collaborations with Harry Stack Sullivan, Erich Fromm and other social scientists over the following decade. The chapter examines the different factors that shaped Thompson's theory of psychoanalysis and clinical practice and the importance she placed on values of equality and openness. In the process, d'Ercole considers the extent to which Thompson's place as a psychoanalytic trailblazer and woman has been neglected.

In the concluding chapter, *Psychoanalysis in the Shadow of Fascism and Genocide: Erich Fromm and the Interpersonal Tradition*, Roger Frie demonstrates that Fromm was one of the few psychoanalysts of the era willing to publicly address the threats posed by the fascism. Fromm's early contribution to the interpersonal perspective in *Psychiatry* (Fromm, 1939) became part of the broader political struggle within psychoanalysis, yet also needs to be read in the wider geopolitical context of the time. For Fromm, the decade of the 1930s spanned his early pioneering work as a member of the Frankfurt School of Social Research in Germany to the creation of the cultural school of psychoanalysis with H. S. Sullivan and K. Horney in the United States. Once in New York, Fromm developed his sociopolitical approach alongside attempts to rescue his Jewish relatives in Germany. The tragic Holocaust history of Fromm's family has been largely overlooked. Frie concludes that there is much to be learned from Fromm's life and work and that his concept of racial narcissism is especially relevant in light of the social and political crises we face today.

Notes

1. Helpful histories of the William Alanson White Institute and its founders can be found in Blechner, M. (2005), Ortmeyer, D. (1995), Perry, H. S. (1982), Shapiro, S. (2017) and Stern, D. (2017).
2. In 1982, in her biography of Sullivan, Helen Swick Perry went so far as to suggest that "No one in America at that time was more advanced than White in his approach to crime" (Perry, 1982, p. 184). Our thanks to Ira Moses for pointing out this quote.

References

Benedict, R. (1938). Continuities and Discontinuities in Cultural Conditioning. *Psychiatry: Journal of the Biology and the Pathology of Interpersonal Relations*, 2, 161–167.

Blechner, M. (2005). The Gay Harry Stack Sullivan: Interactions Between his Life, Clinical Work and Theory. *Contemporary Psychoanalysis*, 41, 1–19.

Brown, J. F. (1938). Freud vs. Marx: Real and Pseudo Problems Distinguished. *Psychiatry: Journal of the Biology and the Pathology of Interpersonal Relations*, 1, 249–255.

Crowley, R. M. (1938). The Courts and Psychiatry. *Psychiatry: Journal of the Biology and the Pathology of Interpersonal Relations*, 1, 265–268.

D'Amore, A. R. T. (1976). *William Alanson White: The Washington years, 1903–1937*. Washington DC: US Department of Health, Education and Welfare.

D'Ercole, A. (in press). *Clara Thompson: The life and work of an American psychoanalyst*. New York: Routledge Press.

Davis, K. (1938). Mental Hygiene and the Class Structure. *Psychiatry: Journal of the Biology and the Pathology of Interpersonal Relations*, 1, 55–65.

Dunham Jr., A. (1938). The Concept of Tension in Philosophy. *Psychiatry: Journal of the Biology and the Pathology of Interpersonal Relations*, 1, 79–120.

Frie, R. (2011). Culture and Context: From Individualism to Situated Experience. In R. Frie and W. J. Coburn (Eds.), *Persons in context: The challenge of individuality in theory and practice* (pp. 3–19). New York: Routledge.

Frie, R. (2013). The Self in Context and Culture. *International Journal of Psychoanalytic Self Psychology*, 8, 505–513.

Frie, R. (2014). Cultural Psychoanalysis: Psychoanalytic Anthropology and the Interpersonal Tradition. *Contemporary Psychoanalysis*, 50, 371–394.

Fromm, E. (1939). The Social Philosophy of "Will Therapy." *Psychiatry: Journal of the Biology and the Pathology of Interpersonal Relations*, 2, 229–237.

Fromm, E. (1941). *Escape from freedom*. New York, NY: Farrar & Rinehart.

Fromm, E. (1947). *Man for himself: An inquiry into psychology and ethics*. Greenwich, CT: Fawcett Premier Books.

Green, M. (1964). *Interpersonal psychoanalysis: Selected papers of Clara Thompson*. New York, NY: Basic Books.

Manson, W. C. (1988). *The psychodynamics of culture: Abram Kardiner and Neo-Freudian anthropology*. New York, NY: Greenwood Press.

Ortmeyer, D. (1995). History of the founders of interpersonal psychoanalysis. In M. Lionells, J. Fiscalini, C. H. Mann, and D. B. Stern (Eds). *Handbook of Interpersonal Psychoanalysis* (pp. 11–30). Hillsdale, NJ: The Analytic Press.

Perry, H.S. (1982). *Psychiatrist of America: The Life Henry Stack Sullivan*. New York, NY: Belknap.

Sapir, E. (1938). Why Cultural Anthropology Needs the Psychiatrist. *Psychiatry: Journal of the Biology and the Pathology of Interpersonal Relations*, 1, 7–12.

Shapiro, S. (2017). History of the William Alanson White Institute Sixty Years after Thompson. *Contemporary Psychoanalysis*, 53, 44–62.

Stern, D. (2017). Introduction. Interpersonal psychoanalysis: History and current status. In D. B. Stern and I. Hirsch (Eds). *The Interpersonal Perspective in Psychoanalysis, 1960s–1990s* (pp. 1–28). New York: Routledge.

Sullivan, H. S. (1938). "Antisemitism." Editorial Notes. *Psychiatry: Journal of the Biology and the Pathology of Interpersonal Relations*, 1, 593–598.

Sullivan, H. S. (1940). Discussion of the Case of Warren Wall. In E. Franklin Frazier. *Negro Youth at the Crossways: Their Personality Development in the Middle States* (pp. 228–234). Washington, D.C.: American Council on Education.

Sullivan, H. S. (1947). Ten years of *Psychiatry*: A statement by the editor. *Psychiatry: Journal of the Biology and the Pathology of Interpersonal Relations*, 10, 433–435.

Sullivan, H. S. (1963). Memorandum on a Psychiatric Reconnaissance. In Martin M. Grossack (Ed.). *Mental Health and Segregation: A Selection of Papers and Some Book Chapters* (pp. 175–179). New York: Springer Pub. Co.

Thompson, C. (1978). Sullivan and Psychoanalysis. *Contemporary Psychoanalysis*, 14, 488–501.

Thompson, C. (1988). Sándor Ferenczi, 1873–1933. *Contemporary Psychoanalysis*, 24, 182–195.

Wake, N. (2011). *Private practices: Harry Stack Sullivan, the science of homosexuality, and American liberalism*. New Brunswick, NJ: Rutgers University Press.

Weigert-Vowinkel, E. (1938). The Cult and Mythology of the Magna Mater from the Standpoint of Psychoanalysis. *Psychiatry: Journal of the Biology and the Pathology of Interpersonal Relations*, 1, 347–378.

White, W. A. (1928). Presidential Address. *Psychoanalytic Review*, 15, 121–131.

White, W. A. (1933). *Crimes and criminals*. New York: Farrar and Rinehart.

William Alanson White Psychiatric Foundation (1938). Mission Statement. *Psychiatry: Journal of the Biology and the Pathology of Interpersonal Relations*, 1, ii.

Winter, S. (1999). *Freud and the institution of psychoanalytic knowledge*. Stanford: Stanford University Press.

Chapter 1

The Roots of Interpersonal Psychoanalysis

Harry S. Sullivan, Interdisciplinary
Inquiry, and Subjectivity[1]

Naoko Wake, Roger Frie, and Pascal Sauvayre

Interpersonal psychoanalysis emerged out of a dialogue between psychiatry, psychoanalysis, and the social sciences during the 1920s and 1930s, which focused on understanding the connection of the individual to culture. Central to this effort was the pioneering work of the American psychiatrist Harry Stack Sullivan (1892–1949). As the social scientist John Dollard remarked, Sullivan was someone "who first made real ... the possibility of a psychiatrist aware of culture" (Dollard, 1935, p. iv). During this formative period, psychiatrists and social scientists from Washington, DC/Baltimore, New Haven, Chicago and beyond gathered at conferences, colloquia, and seminars, driven by an interest in understanding the foundational concept of "life history." This generative interaction reached its height in the late 1930s, when the William Alanson White Foundation published the journal *Psychiatry*, whose aim was to highlight the interdisciplinary collaboration of leading clinicians, scholars, and scientists. The aim of this chapter is to shed light on the emergence of this rich intellectual tradition, highlighting Sullivan's place within it.

Life History and Psychoanalysis

Psychiatry in the 1920s was in an identity crisis, which stemmed from its perceived lack of scientific credibility and professional respectability. In medical communities, it was looked down upon as an immature science at best or, worse, as a non-science. The question of professional respectability was inseparable from this perceived backwardness. In response to these challenges, some psychiatrists used predominantly

DOI: 10.4324/9781003270355-2

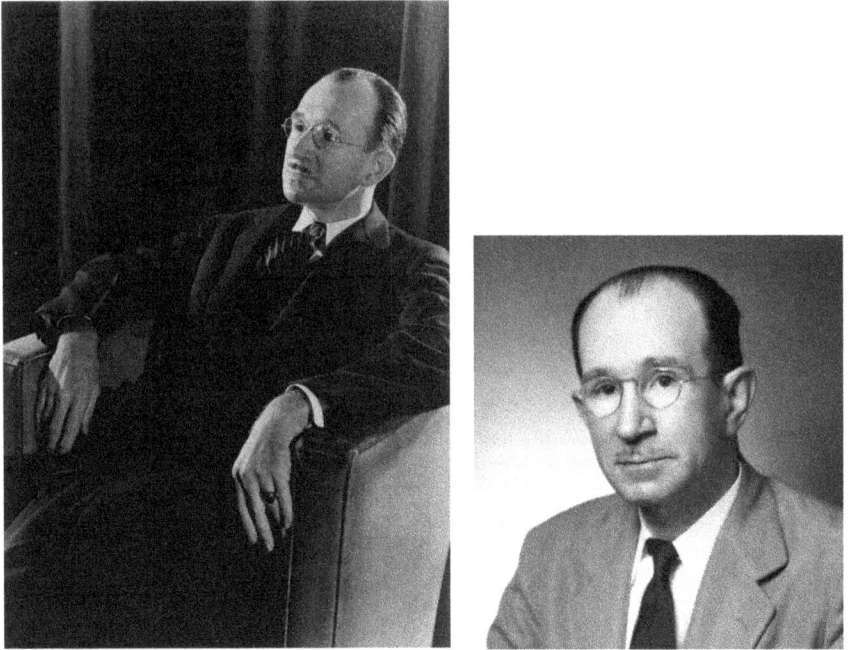

Figure I Harry Stack Sullivan.

biological explanations for mental disorders, a perspective widely prevalent today. Other psychiatrists sought credibility and respectability in a new "science" of the human mind, psychoanalysis, which was becoming popular in the United States following Sigmund Freud's now famous lecture at Clark University in 1909.

Psychoanalysis offered a different set of theories, terms, and therapeutic techniques that embodied the coming of enlightenment, moving beyond the age of ignorance and confusion (see Thompson and Mullahy, 1950; Alexander and Selesnick, 1966; Fancher, 1973). But the majority of American psychiatrists remained suspicious of psychoanalysis because of its idiosyncratic emphasis on the unconscious, the "primitive," and the irrational. They continued to believe that it was crucial for psychiatric medicine to adopt strictly biological and physiological models of explanation. While psychoanalysis might help understand mental problems, it alienated many psychiatrists in the medical profession. In particular, psychoanalysts trained in Europe, many of whom were not medical doctors, posed a threat to the frail confidence of psychiatrists. Psychoanalysis thus generated an ambivalent response from mainstream psychiatry so that by the late 1930s and early 1940s, American psychiatrists began to expel non-medical psychoanalysts from their professional organizations (see Hale, 1995, pp. 141–156, 161–166).

At this time of uncertainty in the profession, the notion of "life history," a foundational concept for a "new psychiatry," began to flourish in psychiatric practice. Many physicians considered the making of a coherent life history the most desirable therapeutic goal. For those who embraced a life history perspective and its interdisciplinary reach across the social sciences, the questionable medical standing of psychoanalysis mattered somewhat less. The intellectual foundation of this new psychiatry was broad and eclectic, as seen in the thinking of Adolf Meyer, a leading figure in the field. Particularly after he cofounded the National Committee for Mental Hygiene (NCMH) in 1911 with an activist and former patient, Clifford W. Beers, Meyer became a driving force in the reform of the profession. Not only did he consider individualized treatment important, he also believed that mental illness should be understood multidimensionally from psychological, biological, and social aspects. Thus, he disagreed with those who narrowly focused on biological factors, while by the same token, he opposed the orthodox Freudians' adherence to a particular set of theories and techniques. The priorities of the followers of the new psychiatry were to obtain data from a person's life with utmost specificity, to understand it in many different contexts, and to highlight the connections between the patients' emotional reactions to experiences, clinical symptoms, and social problems (see Burnham, 1960, pp. 457–465; Grob, 1983, pp. 145, 120–122, 160–166; Lunbeck, 1994, pp. 20–24, 177–181).

Among the paradigms in psychiatry, the new psychiatry was unique in reaching out to other disciplines. Unlike biological and psychoanalytical theorists, psychiatrists in the new psychiatry chose to be inclusive of the natural sciences, social sciences, and humanities in order to create a new discipline—a science of interpersonal relations, as Sullivan called it. The psychiatric researchers of life history constituted a unique group that embraced interdisciplinarity and individual subjectivity in the increasingly specializing field of medicine.

In contrast to new psychiatry, the interest of social scientists in life history came more or less from the opposite direction: from the general to the specific. Going against the predominant interest in statistical methods in sociology, for instance, Dollard in *Criteria for the Life History* (1935) criticized scholars who "simply drop a statistical bucket into the well of [individual] experience and draw it out; they will view their bucketful of data as self-explanatory and not as a part of an individual unified life" (p. 26). What was missing from the statistical approach was contextualization of how experience makes subjective sense to a person:

> After we have "gone cultural" we experience the person as a fragment of a … cultural pattern…. A culture-personality problem can be identified … by observing whether a person is "there" in full emotional reality; if he is not there, then we are dealing with a straight cultural or institutional history. If he is there and we can ask how he feels, then we have a culture-personality problem.
> (Dollard, 1935, p. 5)

In examining culture-personality problems, Dollard used life history to integrate individual, fragmentary, and emotional factors with the cultural and institutional.

This interest in the integration of subjectivity into what was traditionally defined as objective data was not uncommon among social scientists. Indeed, the lack of qualitative analyses in qualitative studies was a vexing concern of American social scientists. Out of this concern emerged a fresh emphasis on the interaction between researchers and their subjects, and on the contexts in which they encountered one another. William I. Thomas in 1928, for instance, discussed what he called "a situational approach," claiming that the increasing interest in the circumstantial factors of social problems had guided sociologists to "life histories, personality documents and records with reference to the concrete trains of experiences" (American Psychiatric Association, 1929, pp. 5–6). Trained at Columbia by Franz Boaz and located at the University of Chicago, the linguist and anthropologist Edward Sapir argued that, in thinking of the link between individuals and collectives, he was "fond of Dr. Sullivan's pet phrase of 'interpersonal relations,'" as the exploration of such relationships helped him to "move forward to a realistic … definition of what is meant by culture and personality" (Sapir, 1937, pp. 863, 870). In 1935, Margaret

Mead reiterated the significance of looking into "inexplicit unformulated ... and uninstitutionalized" aspects of culture, such as child training and family relations, which had been excluded from the issues that ethnographers examined regularly. Moreover, she said, it was crucial that researchers, when collecting information about these "inexplicit" aspects of culture, make "a much more extended entrée into the lives of the people, a much more complete participation in their lives" (Mead, 1935, pp. 7, 9, 15). Mead was not alone in stressing the importance of participant observation in collecting life histories. Harvard anthropologist Florence R. Kluckhohn, for instance, reported in 1940 on her experience of gathering data while she "lived" in a village in New Mexico. She did not reveal that she was an anthropologist, but attempted to obtain information of villagers' real "life-activities" as she assumed the personas of a wife and a storekeeper. Such participatory method would "provide a desirable balance between the ... behavoristic [sic] type of investigation and the type which seeks some measure of insight into the 'meanings' current in the community" (Kluckhohn, 1940, p. 337). All these approaches demanded researchers' attention to concrete, if often fleeting, details, and a fuller involvement in the situation where these details came alive.

Freudian "applied psychoanalysis" had also augmented social scientists' interest in using life history interdisciplinarily (see Manson, 1988). Indeed, the American Sociological Society (ASS) and the American Psychiatric Association (APA) each created a special committee in 1928 and 1927, respectively, to cultivate collaboration between the disciplines. The ASS committee appointed William I. Thomas as a chairman, and Kimball Young and Robert E. Park as its members, suggesting that there was an overlap between people who joined the debate over subjectivity and those who were curious about psychoanalysis (see American Psychiatric Association, 1927, pp. 353–354). Even before the committee was established, there existed a sociological interest in psychoanalysis as seen in Park's *The Principles of Human Behavior* (1915). Published six years after Freud's lecture at Clark University, the book discussed how people are often unconscious of their motives, suggesting the limits of sociological data based on what people could consciously recall in response to sociologists' inquiries. In 1918, William Ogburn similarly used the Freudian concept of "unconsciousness" in his analysis of economy. Following up on his discussion, Thomas Eliot in 1920 discussed the development of a person from an individual to a collective mode of living, using psychoanalytic diagrams of personality proposed by the psychoanalyst Smith Ely Jellifee. Freud's ideas thus offered sociologists a variety of theoretical tools and metaphors with which to explore territories of human life that had been unfamiliar to them and which, despite their importance, might not be easily observable.

What prompted social scientists to explore these unknown territories well before psychoanalysis became the mainstream in American psychiatry? Eliot's assumption about the contrast between youth, immaturity, and foreignness, and the presumed maturity of Western civilization offers a clue. Such an assumption was hardly unique to Eliot. As is clear in the frequent use of the word "primitive" by the era's anthropologists and ethnographers when referring to non-Western societies, one of the shared assumptions in these disciplines was that such research subjects were throwbacks to prehistoric times. Indeed, anthropologists considered it to be an urgent mission to collect data before these non-Western cultures became extinct as a result of being exposed to modernization and Western civilization. Although this did not mean that researchers did not appreciate the characteristics of non-Western societies per se, their value as research subjects lay in their assumed lack of modernity and civilization. Thus Elton Mayo, in 1937, asserted that social maladjustments were rare in a "primitive tribe" because "the passage [from childhood to adulthood] offers no great difficulty." These communities had "established tribal beliefs and the routines, [which would] insure the effective collaboration of the group" in assisting their members' growing up. This was not the case in a more complex, "civilized society." As Freud had discovered, "defective social conditioning" had been causing a wide range of maladjustments including neurosis, promiscuity, and sexual "perversion" (Mayo, 1937, pp. 829–830). The assumption here is that the more a society becomes "civilized," the more problems it begins to suffer. There was a clear parallel made between "underdeveloped" and "developed" personalities on the one hand, and "primitive" and "civilized" societies on the other, thus underlining the colonial and racial narrative ensconced in Freud's thinking (see Gilman, 1985; Brickman, 2003; Frosh, 2013). To better understand the difference drawn between "primitive" and "civilized" societies, and more important, to find scientific solutions to modern problems through examining the difference, the psychoanalytic exploration of the "primitive" seemed indispensable to sociologists.

The "primitive" was not confined to foreign countries; it could be found at home as well. Read Bain, a sociologist who played a crucial role in the introduction of Freud to American social scientists, pointed to an increasing number of "psychopaths" in the United States. Refusing the idea that a person can be born to be sick, Bain asserted that "psychoses" such as "the homosexual syndrome" was a "masculine protest" against "women's clubs aping men and [men's] clubs." According to Bain, then, men who frequent "psychotic groups [such as] gangs [and] homosexual colonies" might be trying to escape pressures brought about by changes in modern society, such as increasing rights for women (Bain, 1936, pp. 208–212). In addition to his rejection of feminism and his understanding of homosexuality as one of the ills of civilization, it is noteworthy that Bain, like Mayo, reiterated the contrast between the "primitive" and "civilized." Among social scientists influenced by Freud, a dualistic thinking that placed Western civilization, complexity, and maturity in contrast with savagery, simplicity, and immaturity of non-Westerners was prevalent. As modern society grew complex, there emerged a gap between those who were better adjusted to the complexity and those who were less adjusted, and it was social scientists' responsibility to understand the latter—the "simple," "primitive," and "immature" in a developed society.

This dualistic model brought social scientists near their "exotic" research subjects, at least as much as it created a distance between researchers and their subjects. Many psychoanalysts and social scientists were intrigued by cultures and personalities that seemed to offer a counterpoint to modernity (see Mead, 1932, chap. 10). While these points of reference were often romanticized (for example, "primitive" societies were deemed to be "preserving" human nature in its bare form), these cultural "others" could also be somewhat uncanny, especially when they were found within modernity. Criminals, delinquents, psychopaths, and perverts—all of whom were popular subjects of 1920s social sciences—seemed to represent just the kind of problems that modern, urban, and diverse America must confront. What was unique to the era's social scientists' response to these "others" was their embrace of—or their attempt to embrace—the subjectivity of both the researcher and the subject, which distinctively separated them from their predecessors for whom the objectivity of their knowledge remained unquestioned. Medical and social scientists, though from different paths, reached the same conclusion that life history was a method that opened up a place for both human uncertainty and scientific clarity. In turn, the work of scientists in the life history cohort created an opening for a kind of science that resisted systematized explanation in order to understand lived complexity. Perhaps the truly striking development in the life history method was its cross-disciplinary roots.

Bridging Psychiatry and Sociology

The APA's and the ASS's committees on interdisciplinary collaboration sponsored a series of conferences called the Colloquium on Personality Investigation, in 1928 and 1929, creating perhaps the era's most important interdisciplinary forum. The ASS contingent included people from the Freud-influenced group, among them Ernest Burgess, Elton Mayo, Harold Lasswell, and Edward Sapir, in addition to the committee members who constituted the core of the life history cohort (and notably, Clifford Shaw as well). The APA representatives included William Alanson White as a chairman and Harry Stack Sullivan as a secretary of the committee, along with psychiatrists such as David Levy, Lawson Lowrey, James S. Plant, and William Healy, all of whom were chief figures of the new psychiatry. In addition, there was Lawrence K. Frank from the Laura Spelman Rockefeller Memorial Foundation and the Social Science Research Council as a sponsor of the colloquium. It was during these colloquia that some of the main concepts of life history were articulated, which in turn revealed how researchers of the era grappled with the meaning of subjectivity in science. Many scientists who attended these colloquia did not see subjectivity as simply individualistic, but rather as embedded in relations with "others." With this goal, scientists at the colloquia elaborated three main and interrelated components of the life history method: "personality," "participant observation," and "social psychiatry."

One of these components, personality, appeared in Park's 1928 preliminary statement on the colloquium: the psychiatrists' "opportunity to study personalities in hospitals, gives them access to aspects of human nature that are not accessible to the sociologists." Indeed, the concept of personality emerged in participants' discussion as an important bridge between sociological and medical thinking. Mark A. May, a social psychologist, fleshed out the concept of personality, stating that it was "the net result of your social interaction" and that personality types, "if there are such, are the result as well as the cause of different kinds of ... social interaction" (APA, 1930, p. 80).

Intrigued by these dynamic definitions, Sullivan asked May to further explain what he meant by personality types. Their exchange illuminates a key intersection of medical and social scientific notions of personality:

> MAY: By types [of personality], I mean types of responses. Therefore, personality is not something that is constant and carried around with you, but personality changes as you go from one type of social group to another. These changes depend entirely upon what goes on between you and the other members of the group....
>
> SULLIVAN: I am reaching for your idea which coincides with mine insofar as I stress the notion that interpersonal relations are invariably interpersonal; that the observer does not sit upon an ivory tower and gaze down at strange objects performing below him, but instead performs with them.
>
> (APA, 1930, pp. 80–82)

Here, what May described as a person in a changing social setting was redefined as "interpersonal relations" by Sullivan, suggesting that in his definition, interpersonal relationships included not merely more than one person, but also social contexts in which an encounter between individuals occurred. Because of this inclusiveness, Edward Sapir would later see a "good meeting ground" for psychiatrists and social scientists in the concept of interpersonal relations (Sapir, 1937, p. 862). Perhaps such recognition by social scientists pushed Sullivan to use it as a key term in his theory in the coming years.

There are other ideas embedded in this exchange that became important both in Sullivan's interpersonal theory of mental illness and in the method of life history. For one, May's statement touched on what was to become one of Sullivan's unique theses: the idea that a person has a unique personality independent of the environment is "illusory" because a person cannot be scientifically isolated from his/her interactions with others. Although May did not argue that individual personality is illusory, he came close when he said that a personality was not constant and could not be carried from one situation to another. Moreover, Sullivan's discussion of the role of the scientist in this exchange corresponded with the concept of "participant observation" that scientific interviewers are participants, with their interviewees, in the process of collecting life histories. Similar to the "interpersonal relation," the concept of participant observation was rooted in his clinical practice at Sheppard and Enoch Pratt Hospital; now it began to take new root in the interdisciplinary community. Surely Sullivan at Sheppard-Pratt understood that he could not perform his duties well as an interviewer if he remained in an ivory tower. In this exchange with May, then, Sullivan can be seen as discovering a tie between the best of his clinical practice and social scientific inquiries. More importantly, "participant observation" became a reminder that scientists were not exempt from subjectivity. This worked against the dualistic distinction between interviewers and interviewees.

Yet another key concept shaped during the colloquia, that of the "social psychiatrist," illuminated the impact of the social sciences on psychiatry. Following the pattern of reform embraced by the new psychiatry, social psychiatrists were expected to excel in understanding mental illness in social contexts. Not surprisingly, psychiatrists at the colloquia proposed a plan to change the curriculum in medical education. Taking note of the lack of dependable treatment, for example, Sullivan argued that in the future, those who would find solutions to mental problems were "social psychiatrists," who, in his definition, were trained in "a good deal of what you [social scientists] have learned" (APA, 1929, pp. 60–61). Some participants suggested that, in light of this, there should be an exchange of professors between the fields: a sociologist lectures in a class on psychiatry at a medical school, a psychiatrist teaches in a course on economics, and so on. These opinions gained further momentum in the second colloquium, when educational reform became a focal point once again. Speaking for sociologists, for example, Ernest Burgess argued that students in the field should work with psychiatrists and psychoanalysts in a graduate course on life history. But Sullivan felt that Burgess's moderate plan did not go far enough: instead of making an exchange program in graduate school, Sullivan insisted on interdisciplinary "departments in which general information rather than [the] highly specialized is the principle" (APA, 1930, pp. 137–138). These departments, because of their focus on undergraduate education, would encourage "people [to] get a good deal of knowledge without too rigid crystallization of ideas" (APA, 1930, p. 140). This went beyond a plan for interdisciplinary collaboration. This was a plea for a new field integrating existing areas of expertise.

Sullivan's proposal to create a new department in a university stimulated lively discussion among the colloquium's participants, suggesting the extent (and the limit) of their idea of multidisciplinary collaboration. Harold Lasswell, then a young political scientist and just back from a trip to Europe, during which he had met such psychoanalysts as Alfred Adler, Gregory Zilboorg, Sandor Ferenczi, and Wilhelm Stekel, was supportive of Sullivan; to create "a grand department of personality study" would be desirable (Lasswell, 1928). On the other hand, Lasswell expressed his reservation as well, suggesting that this plan might belong to a distant future. The more immediate concern should be to create opportunities for researchers from different disciplines to learn about each other's interests. This moderate approach to cross-disciplinary collaboration, rather than something as dramatic as Sullivan's, was preferred by most participants, even those who clearly shared Sullivan's frustration with the lack of psychiatric education at medical schools.

Interdisciplinary Scientists at Work

By the late 1920s, various endeavors for interdisciplinary collaboration were under way. For example, Harold Lasswell launched his research on personality at a mental hospital soon after the second colloquium, the result of which was published as *Psychopathology and Politics* in 1930. Lasswell and Sullivan joined the seminar called "Culture and Personality" at Yale University in 1932 and 1933, funded through Lawrence Frank at the Social Science Research Council and organized by Edward Sapir. In Chicago, the impact of life history and psychoanalytic methods remained strong, producing some of the best-known sociological studies of urban slums, gangs, and immigrant communities under Robert E. Park and Ernest Burgess's initiative. In 1937, sociologists Allison Davis and John Dollard began a case study of "personality development from a combined psychological and cultural point of view," using African American children in New Orleans and Natchez, Mississippi, as their subjects (Davis and Dollard, 1940, p. xii). Based on the discussion in the colloquia, Sullivan also designed a new curriculum in psychiatric postgraduate education. When he established the Washington School of Psychiatry in 1936, he invited social scientists, including Harold Lasswell, Erich Fromm, and Ruth F. Benedict, as lecturers. These social scientists contributed to *Psychiatry*, an interdisciplinary journal that Sullivan and the publications committee of the William Alanson White Psychiatric Foundation founded in 1938. The journal published articles from psychiatrists, psychoanalysts, and diverse scholars in the social sciences and humanities and it remained interdisciplinary throughout Sullivan's lifetime. In 1947, Sullivan reviewed 350 items that had appeared in the journal during its first decade, and found that the 197 authors of these items included, apart from mental health professionals, 19 sociologists, 13 anthropologists, 7 political scientists, 6 educators, 4 social workers, 3 lawyers, 2 philosophers, and 2 historians (see Sullivan, 1947, pp. 433–435). Along with these developments, Alfred H. Stanton, a psychiatrist who would work with Sullivan at the Chestnut Lodge Hospital in the 1940s, and Morris S. Schwartz, a University of Chicago sociologist, collaborated in the 1930s on research on the impact of the institutional environment on psychiatric patients. Their work resulted in a landmark sociological study, *The Mental Hospital*, published in 1954. Finally, there were conferences in 1934 and 1947 on interdisciplinary collaboration in the study of culture and personality. These conferences were outgrowths of the personality colloquia and were attended by anthropologists, psychologists, and psychiatrists (see Sargent and Smith, 1949).

Sullivan's plan to transform the society and science that lacked a full understanding of the mentally ill began a new phase in the 1930s. One of the earliest signs of this interdisciplinary program was the establishment of his interpersonal theory of mental illness. While Sullivan's use of the word *interpersonal* remained somewhat fluid during the 1920s, it was clearly the most important concept in his theory by the mid-1930s. During the 1920s, he often used the adjective *interpersonal* interchangeably with *societal* (see for instance, Sullivan, 1929a, pp. 108–109). Many of his unpublished manuscripts did not include the term, but instead employed descriptive explanations such as "[a person] govern[s] himself in accordance with the wishes of others" (Sullivan, 1926, p. 22) and "cultural symbols ... are derived entirely from events including other persons" (Sullivan, 1926, p. 28). In other cases, he used a compound word, *inter-personal*, not the singular term *interpersonal* (Sullivan, 1929b, p. 702). But in the mid-1930s, he came to use the adjective *interpersonal* more regularly in combination with relation, making it a key concept in his writing (see, for example, Sullivan, 1934). As he settled on this term, his theoretical scope was adjusted accordingly. In the early 1930s, his writing came to include a systematic discussion of stages of "normal" personality development, departing from his earlier focus on mental "abnormality." Similarly, in his published writing on interpersonal relations, the issue of homo-sexuality was not clearly demarcated as such but rather folded into the developmental theory of homosexuality.

Personal Psychopathology and Homosexuality

This is nowhere better seen than in the pages of *Personal Psychopathology* (1972), a book written between 1929 and 1933. Here, Sullivan offered his first comprehensive theory of personality devel-opment (which would remain an essential feature of his thought) in which he embedded a critique of homophobia that he had been developing for some time. In this, his first monograph, Sullivan made it clear that his subject was not a theory of mental disorders, but one involving "typical courses of events" consisting of "matters of common experience" (1972, p. 2)—a life process in general. Thus, he discussed developmental stages, beginning with "infancy," then moving through "childhood," the "juvenile era," "pre-adolescence," "adolescence," and "adulthood." In each of the stages, development is defined by the interpersonal processes involved. For instance, an infant is born into a "primary group" that consists of two people—an infant and a mother. In this primary group, an infant develops "facil-ities for communication," (p. 11) such as smiling, crying, and tem-per tantrums. These facilities are responses to a mother's emotional conditions: when she is happy, the infant feels secure; when she is nervous, her baby develops insecurity. This tight emotional synchronization he called "empathy" remains an important factor in any interpersonal relation throughout life. Infancy ends when "the young one begins to acquire the spoken language of his people" roughly at the age of eighteen months (p. 29). In "childhood," with the appearance of articulate speech, a child's personality comes to be exposed to sociocultural factors, and a "certain … type of ideals and ambitions" emerges in a child's consciousness. A young one becomes a "creature of culture" in childhood, Sullivan concluded (pp. 40–41).

In the "juvenile era," a child enters a "secondary group" which includes people beyond immediate family members, such as teachers and classmates in grade school so that "others" come to carry more importance. At this stage, however, the socialization with others is primarily egocentric. A child shows an appreciation of the needs of others only when they are favorable to his or her own interests (p. 42). In "preadolescence," the egocentric character of a child's sociality subsides with the emergence of the need for an intimate playmate of similar age. It becomes more important to contribute to the pleasure of the other when contributions to the self-esteem of a "chum" matter more than the satisfaction of one's self-interest. In this close association with a chum, "peculiarities of the home life … tend to lose their … effectiveness because they fall into unfavorable comparison with similar factors in the home life of the other." Thus, the chum relationship is the beginning of a "social world," where conflicts brought from family relationships may be resolved as a "result of … new experience toward a rational integration." Consequently, the likelihood that members of a well-integrated social world grow healthily is high (pp. 164–167). In "adolescence," a need for an intimate interpersonal relation is directed toward a person of the opposite sex. When one achieves a stable relation involving another person of the opposite sex, in which "sexual drives, desires, or needs" are resolved, this person enters into "adulthood" (p. 44).

In *Personal Psychopathology*, all the stage markers in personality development are defined as changes in interpersonal relations. It is also obvious that the sociocultural factors that had an impact on personality development were more than those related to sexuality. Reflecting the expansion of his theoretical scope, which was pushed by his collaboration with social scientists, Sullivan's discussion in

Personal Psychopathology included a range of interpersonally and socially constructed events.

Embedded in this scheme, however, was Sullivan's emphasis on the importance of broadening the realm of socially acceptable sexual relationships. He noted, for instance, the significance of chumship which, in his definition, was a close friendship between children of the same sex, insuring a sense of belonging that helped a child find a place in a larger group of same-sex friends. This larger group, sometimes called a "gang," often manifested sexual intimacies such as "mutual masturbation … and homosexual procedures" (p. 165). Contradicting mainstream psychiatric theories that defined this as a "deleterious" and "unfortunate … homosexual stage" (p. 170), Sullivan argued that these expressions of homoeroticism strengthened a bond within the group and helped its members to adjust to heterosexual relationships later in their lives:

> I have had opportunity to study one community in regard to the alleged evil consequences of these factors.… In this community—a large number of early adolescents participated in overt homosexual activities during the gang age. Most of them progressed … to the customary heteroerotic interest in later adolescence. Some of the few boys in this community who were excluded from the gangs as a result of their powerful inhibitions, who missed participation in community homosexual play, did not progress to satisfactory heterosexual development (p. 171).

Here, Sullivan's assertion was that homosexual experiences at a young age were crucial for heterosexual maturity in later years. Such a developmental conceptualization of homosexuality was challenged by many of his Sheppard-Pratt patients who experienced homosexuality in its own right. Even so, he pointedly argued that, in a sexually rigid culture (such as modern American culture), "there is generally sufficient personal frustration … [to necessitate] sexual fantasy with almost any symbols" (p. 163), including those of a homosexual nature. On the one hand, his discussion of sexual problems would take the form of a more general analysis of interpersonal relations. On the other, his recognition of the importance of same-sex intimacy and his critique of homophobia are palpable between the lines.

Only in moderate tone and language did Sullivan in *Personal Psychopathology* criticize the limited social acceptance of homosexuality. In the U.S. general population, the proportion of people who "completed the evolution to the state of adulthood," an intimate relationship with a partner of the opposite sex, was "not very great" (pp. 43–44). Because of the popular belief that "woman is declassed [when she has] sexual intercourse with a man, before having married him, ... a turning to the autoerotic or the homoerotic types of interests" was common (p. 194). If these common interests were socially accepted, the benefit could be immense. Indeed, as Sullivan argued, "homoerotic interests in the female ... encounter little social disapproval; in fact, there is almost no attention given the erotic elements accompanying such relationship." Compared with her male counterpart, a female homosexual achieved "an easier adaptation to her role" in her adult life (p. 258). Nevertheless, there remained the fact that his emphasis was framed by a developmental theory that assumed that same-sex sexual relationships were not part of a complete adulthood. The question of what should be done in a society that did not allow a majority of its members to achieve full maturity was left unarticulated. This was a departure from his recognition at Sheppard-Pratt that, because homosexual relationships are common, people with homosexual conflicts should encourage society to better accept them rather than wasting their time trying to grow out of homoeroticism.

Even this modified approach to homosexuality elicited his colleagues' reservations about *Personal Psychopathology* as a scientific monograph. Edward Sapir used it as a textbook in his culture and personality seminar at Yale University, and its members thought that it was too centered on psychoanalysis, suffering from Freud's apparently outbalanced emphasis on the importance of libido. If this suggested an uneasy status that both Freud and sexuality occupied in American science, the title of the book fueled a rumor that the work was Sullivan's autobiography. Eventually, Sullivan withdrew the book from publication, noting that the monograph was only "privately circulated" (ix). In this way, his attempt to include his subjectivity in science was circumscribed, even as it was embedded in his professional concern for interpersonal relationships. A scientist's subjectivity, especially that related to sexuality, was denied a role in scientific theory.

After the two colloquia on personality investigation in 1928 and 1929, then, Sullivan embarked on more clear-cut research programs that would not raise questions of subjectivity—at least not in the way that *Personal Psychopathology* did. In 1932, he joined Sapir's Yale seminar, making it a habit to travel to New Haven once a week. By then, Sullivan was a close friend of Sapir, who had been at the University of Chicago and had just relocated to Yale University's Institute of Human Relations. In addition to attending seminars, Sullivan often went to Sapir's second house on a New Hampshire farm during summers, where Sapir spent time with his second wife, Jean, and his children (Perry, 1972, p. 335). Through Sapir, Sullivan became acquainted with rising social scientists such as John Dollard and Hortense Powdermaker, as well as Mark A. May, with whom Sullivan had had a (aforementioned) discussion on the social context of interpersonal relations at the colloquium (Johnson, 1952).

Race and Racism

This group of social scientists offered Sullivan both intellectual inspiration and institutional grounds from which he could take leave of the sensitive subject of homosexuality and develop an apparently more mainstream science of interpersonal relations. The group's research programs in 1932 and 1933 mirrored some of the recognizable trends in the era's scholarship, while they also indicated a new direction of social scientific studies. Dollard, who was first appointed as a fellow and then as an assistant director of the seminar, had been working on psychotic behavior from sociological standpoints. His patron Ernest Burgess at the University of Chicago praised Dollard's all-around training in "statistical, case-study, cultural and psychoanalytic techniques" (Burgess, 1939, p. 373), suggesting Dollard's already strong interest in an interdisciplinary approach to life history. Dollard's interdisciplinarity would soon materialize in a series of works, *Criteria for the Life History* (1935), *Caste and Class in Southern Town* (Dollard, 1937), and *Children of Bondage* (1940). Further, in his report on the status of psychological studies of personality in Germany, Dollard took note of Ernest Kretschmer's theory positing that "lower" and "primitive" stages of cultural function appear in "higher" and "civilized" men, especially among schizophrenics. Here again was the parallel between primitiveness and schizophrenia. Along with these, Hortense Powdermaker's study of an African American community in Mississippi seemed to have a considerable impact on Sullivan's intellectual career. In her engagement with what she called the first anthropological study of a contemporary community in the United States, Powdermaker collaborated with black scholars Charles S. Johnson and E. Franklin Frazier at Fisk University. Sullivan reviewed her proposal for a Social Science Research Council fellowship to support her research, which helped him to shape his own research agendas (Perry, 1982, pp. 347–358).

By the late 1930s, Sullivan was thus working on several projects about a great range of sociocultural contexts associated with mental problems. In a 1938 article, he mentioned "reductions in employment, reductions in the standard of living, and damage to the prestige of collective national, racial, regional and class symbols" as possible causes of stress and conflict. Also, he noted that psychiatrists needed to place these factors "in proper relation to the total historical evolution of conflicting values" (1938a). To substantiate these statements, Sullivan extended his examinations of social problems, some of which were a direct outgrowth of the Yale seminar. In particular, his interest in race problems in the United States became so prominent in his research that it might be said that his focus shifted from homophobia to racism, at least in his public discussion. In 1937 and 1938, for example, he collaborated with Johnson and Frazier, who were by then investigating personality problems among young blacks under the sponsorship of the American Council of Education (ACE). Sullivan's role in these studies was to talk to black youths to determine the impact of their racial, class, and geographical environment on their personalities (Sullivan, 1940; 1941). Frazier had been focusing on the population in the middle states, while Johnson's research had been about the Deep South. Sullivan served as a consultant to both, interviewing no fewer than twenty African American youths, mostly in Washington, DC, and Memphis, Tennessee, so as to offer psychiatric insight into the influence of racial tensions on these individuals' personality development. He drew a couple of interesting conclusions that suggested the new direction of his research. He noted, for example, that he did not find any "typical Negro characteristics" among his informants:

The tragedy of the Negro in America seems to be chiefly a matter of culturally determined attitudes in the whites.... However, when ... the techniques of intensive study of interpersonal relations have been substituted for those of a detached and generally preoccupied professional man, the presumptively "typically Negro" performances have been resolved into particular instances of the "typically human."

(Sullivan, 1940, p. 233)

Sullivan saw, for instance, that "fear" of whites, widespread among African Americans in the South, was related to the "great violence" done toward them, especially lynching. He did not attribute this fear to African Americans' race. He made a similar observation about young blacks in Washington, DC. He found that most of them were struggling with deep "rage" against whites, but was quick to point out that this rage resulted from inequality between blacks and whites in the city, not from a racial temperament (Sullivan, 1941, pp. 329–331). In life histories of his black informants, then, Sullivan found unambiguous evidence of social construction of so-called natural categories.

In this project for the ACE, Sullivan also discovered that this field of research—race relationships in the United States—was an ideal arena in which to apply the method of participant observation. Without doubt, he was aware of the limits of communication between himself, a white man, and African American individuals. One of his descriptions of an interview with an "outstanding" leader of the black community, for example, illuminates Sullivan's approach to the distance between the races:

I think that this leader ... progressed in our acquaintanceship only from a distrust of my motives, through a distrust of my judgment, to a vague wondering if I might actually be a detached observer without blinding preconceptions and group loyalties hostile to him and his people. He seemed to me one of the loneliest of men; a well-trained professional man of rather keen sensitivity, isolated in the nexus of several fields of hostility, so driven by some complex of motives (which proved mostly inaccessible to me) (1941, p. 330).

Here, Sullivan admitted that there were certain things about the interviewee that he could not grasp. Unlike his earlier, relentless insistence at Sheppard-Pratt that patients reveal all things possible to him, Sullivan let this informant remain "inaccessible." But he did not dismiss the value of information obtained. Instead, he drew the conclusion that the interviewee's lack of openness indicated the serious impact of racial antagonism, in contrast to an internal pathology. Apparently, such a critique of race problems was far easier for Sullivan to publish than was his protest against homophobia. On the one hand, race problems allowed him to develop ideas that mattered to him: a critique of "culturally determined attitudes" that caused "tragedy" in those who were discriminated against; a better understanding of the fear of being open and honest, prevalent among minorities (Sullivan, 1940, p. 233). On the other hand, he did not have to worry about being seen as overly subjectively involved in his science, as he did at Sheppard-Pratt and in *Personal Psychopathology*. With patients suffering from homosexual conflicts, he insisted that he know everything because he felt that he could and he must; with African Americans, he was accepting of the fact that there was "inaccessible" information, things that would remain unknown to him. His subjects were racial minorities, not sexual ones, and his whiteness was obvious in a way his sexuality was not. This made it easy for him to claim scientific objectivity.

The study of race also taught him how to discuss sexuality in a more mainstream, less controversial way. In his observation of a sixteen-year-old black boy in Washington, DC, for instance, Sullivan revealed his sense of what he deemed a positive attitude toward sex among African Americans. This informant said that he had masturbated with his younger brother when they were small kids, seemingly without the feelings of guilt that Sullivan had seen too commonly among his white patients at Sheppard-Pratt. The informant also claimed that he had sexual intercourse with girls and talked to his father about it when he discovered that one of these girls gave him a sexually transmitted disease. His father did not punish him, but instead helped him to get the "necessary treatments" and showed him "how to relieve" himself. In response to these details of life history that he hardly encountered in his clinical practice, Sullivan argued, "Vividly outstanding factors in ... many Negro family groups are superficially identical with those which in whites eventuate in arrest of heterosexual development and thus to obligate homosexual or bisexual patterns of behavior" (1940, p. 230). Here, "outstanding factors" in black families were a recognition of sex as an important part of human life. These factors were identical to white families' only "superficially," because whites turned the recognition of sex into strict sexual inhibitions. In this contrast between the races, then, Sullivan's critique of homophobia took a more general, recognizable form of an examination of white Americans' limited approach to sex and to white fantasies about black sexuality.

This approach made sense in the intellectual climate of the 1930s. By the end of the decade, it was not unusual for physicians, psychologists, and sociologists to argue that seeing masturbation as a cause of mental problems was misguided. In addition, as seen in studies of researchers such as Powdermaker, Sullivan, and Dollard, a cultural, rather than biological, understanding of race was becoming the norm among progressive medical and social scientists, though this understanding was still circumscribed by the limit of their liberal thoughts. In particular, African Americans in the South attracted these scientists' interest as "others" who were nevertheless "within" American society—"American primitive(s)" who "promised both abnormality and authenticity" as research subjects (Rose, 2005, p. 337). In Sullivan's discussion, it is not difficult to see that he benefited from both the supposed abnormality and the authenticity of blacks. His characterization of African Americans as sexually "permissive" can be seen as being connected to the racist belief that all African Americans are "promiscuous." Indeed, he asserted, "there are many definitely promiscuous [black] people" and "this laxity arises from ... a permissive culture." But he also disagreed with the misconception that all blacks are promiscuous when he wrote: "I have to speak ... against using them [African Americans] as scapegoats for our [whites'] unacceptable impulses; the fact that they are ... poorly adapted to our historic puritanism is really too naïve a basis for projecting most of our privately condemned faults upon them" (1940, p. 234). This statement recognized that whites' fear of sex had indeed been projected on blacks, illuminating how African Americans were a "subject" close enough and, at the same time, different enough for white scientists to explore. This mixture of fascination, respect, and prejudice lay beneath Sullivan's discussion of African Americans' attitude toward sex. It was precisely this mixture that made it easier for him to discuss sexuality within the context of race problems rather than as the problem of homophobia.

Compared with white homosexual men then, blacks were not close enough to Sullivan's subjectivity to force him to probe how it felt to be stigmatized. He could "participate" in African American life histories, highlighting injustice of both racial and sexual kinds, while keeping his own personal subjectivity at arms' length. In concluding his argument, he stressed that white Americans must "cultivate a humanistic rather than a paternalistic attitude" to blacks (1940, p. 233–234). Reading this statement, no one would have wondered if he made a similar point about homosexual individuals (which he did at Sheppard-Pratt). This was because there was no hint of the scientist's homosexuality and subjectivity in this statement, even though the discussion was about sexuality.

It is ironic that, right around this time, he suggested that his white male friends sleep with black women to become free sexually. Moreover, less than two years after he drew the conclusion about the need for a more racially aware attitude toward African Americans, he was involved in the psychiatric screening for the Selective Service, which accentuated racism. The lack of subjective involvement had its consequences, which were most conspicuous in the ways in which Sullivan interacted with African American researchers in the 1930s. Working with Johnson, for example, Sullivan consistently arranged meetings in his office either in New York City or Washington, DC. When Johnson asked Sullivan to visit him in Nashville, Sullivan sent an apologetic letter noting that his "alleged financing program has made no material progress [and he] see[s] no immediate possibility" of traveling. This prompted Johnson to reiterate that he would make "available a fund for travel and expenses." Such an uneven relationship persisted even after the completion of the research. In 1939, Johnson recommended an African American student at Fisk to meet with Sullivan, so that the student could be trained in psychiatric techniques of personality study. It took Sullivan three and half months to respond. When he eventually did, he filled his letter with details of his busy schedule and his suggestion that the student read his soon to be published lecture notes rather than attending his lectures at the Washington School of Psychiatry. It is not clear if Sullivan thought about the impact of inviting a black student to an all-white institute. Regardless, Johnson's response was respectful, acknowledging "the pressure on you" that must have caused "the long delay." But with two more months without a word from Sullivan, Johnson wrote another letter to urge him to set up an appointment with the student. Yet another month passed, and Johnson's next letter suggested that the student follow Sullivan to Cincinnati where he was scheduled to attend a conference. There was no indication that Sullivan ever responded to this rather urgent plea (Johnson, 1938–1940). His critique of racism, which he put out in public forcefully, did not seem to shape his person-to-person interactions with his black colleagues.

Despite this standoffishness, which might or might not have been a sign of the limit of Sullivan's race awareness but was most likely interpreted as such by Johnson, their collaboration opened up an arena for a range of skills and expertise to come together, putting psychiatry at the center of the interdisciplinary scholarship (Rose, 2005). Sullivan's theory of mental illness made a notable contribution to the new psychiatry and the mental hygiene movement as well. One important feature in *Personal Psychopathology* and his articles in the 1930s was his assertion of a possibility for substantive change in a personality throughout preadolescence and adolescence. This was a positive view, especially when it was applied to mental illness, because it suggested a hope for recovery even at relatively advanced ages. In addition, Sullivan's specialty since his Sheppard-Pratt days in the eyes of many had been schizophrenia. Schizophrenia was among the most serious of mental illnesses, and it continued to be the single largest diagnosis given to inmates at state institutions throughout the 1920s and 1930s. Sullivan's optimism, combined with his ever-expanding emphasis on sociocultural factors, pointed toward the hope that even people with schizophrenia could be cured, if society were different. Increasingly, it was his belief that society could dramatically improve through intellectual and institutional innovations. And he had many plans to change medical education; there were issues other than race to be included in the interdisciplinary research programs. These tasks came to occupy a considerable part of Sullivan's professional life.

Innovative and Interdisciplinary Education

As seen in the discussion at the colloquia, the reform of medical education was a widely shared concern among psychiatrists, especially those who supported the new psychiatry. In the early 1930s, Frankwood E. Williams and William A. White—both representatives of the National Institute of Mental Health—and Sullivan, fresh from his success at the colloquia, helped create a Joint Committee on Psychiatric Education for the APA (Williams, 1928). Sullivan's plan for a medical school curriculum was demanding. In the freshman year, lectures on cultural anthropology, sociology, economics, political science, literature, art, and history would be offered. In the second year, students would be required to examine their own life histories with their supervisors (Sullivan, 1931). In their third and fourth years, students would begin "supervised contact with carefully selected clinical material," allowing them to practice participant observation and life history method in a quasi-clinical setting (Sullivan, 1939, p. 276). It is apparent that Sullivan's curriculum was nothing if not radically different from the standard. Most medical schools during the 1920s and 1930s offered courses on biology, chemistry, physics, anatomy, physiology, pathology, and pharmacology in the first years of medical education, but almost never included the social sciences and humanities (Rothstein, 1987; Haller Jr., 1994).

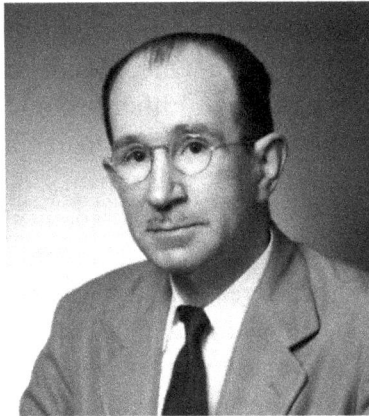

Figure 2 Edward Sapir.

Sullivan's proposal found the first opportunity for institutional application at the Washington School of Psychiatry, established with Sullivan as a head of the Division of Psychiatry, psychiatrist Ernest Hadley as a chair of the Division of Biological Sciences, and Edward Sapir as a director of the Division of Social Sciences. Soon after the school was established, an arrangement was made with the Washington-Baltimore Psychoanalytic Society for its members to take courses in psychoanalysis at the school. Moreover, as Charles S. Johnson's recommendation of his student at Fisk University suggested, the school was open to social science students who desired to learn psychiatry (Sullivan, 1938b). The class titled "Non-Clinical Psychoanalysis" consisted of roundtable presentations: Sullivan's "Psychoanalysis and Social Sciences," Ruth Benedict's "Cultural Anthropology," Randolph Paul's "Taxation," Harold Lasswell's "Political Sciences," E. M. Jellinek's "Statistics," Howard Rowland's "Sociology," and Tom Gill's "Literature" (see William Alanson White Psychiatric Foundation, 1939, pp. 476, IV). Additionally, Erich Fromm offered lectures in the field of social psychology (Friedman, 2013, p. 87). This list of presentations mirrored the lineup of articles and authors in *Psychiatry*. In the journal's inaugural issue from 1938, Sullivan explained that psychiatry "is becoming a science that is fundamental ... to research into almost any aspect of people and interpersonal relations, broadly conceived" (Sullivan, 1938b, p. 141).

The 1930s was thus a time when psychoanalytically "oriented," if not "trained," psychiatrists such as White and Sullivan were influential in both psychiatry and psychoanalysis. They worked together with leading psychoanalysts such as Clara Thompson, Karen Horney, Erich Fromm, and Frieda Fromm-Reichmann to support the consideration of social and cultural factors. In this climate, Sullivan continued to promote his theory of interpersonal relations at the Washington School of Psychiatry and in the journal *Psychiatry*. This process of cross-disciplinary learning and practice reached fruition in 1943, when Sullivan, Fromm, Fromm-Reichman, and Thompson joined with David Rioch, a research neurophysiologist, and Janet Rioch, a pediatrician, to establish the William Alanson White Institute of Psychiatry, Psychoanalysis and Psychology in New York, named in honor of White who died in 1937.

Note

1. Readers can find more information in N. Wake (2011). *Private Practices,* Chapter 3, pp. 86–115, from which parts of this essay have been adapted.

References

Alexander, F. and Selesnick, S. (1966). *The history of psychiatry: An evaluation of psychiatric thought and practice from prehistoric times to the present.* New York: Harper & Row.

American Psychiatric Association. (1927). Proceedings: Report of the council meeting, June 3. *American Journal of Psychiatry,* 84, 353–354.

American Psychiatric Association. (1928). Proceedings: Report of the committee on statistics. *American Journal of Psychiatry,* 85, 370–372.

American Psychiatric Association. (1929). *Proceedings: First colloquium on personality investigation.* Ann Arbor: MI: University of Michigan Press.

American Psychiatric Association. (1930). *Proceedings: Second colloquium on personality investigation.* Ann Arbor: MI: University of Michigan Press.

Bain, R. (1936). Sociology and psychoanalysis. *American Sociological Review,* 1, 203–316.

Brickman, C. (2003). *Aboriginal populations in the mind.* New York, NY: Columbia University Press.

Burgess, E. (1939). The influence of Sigmund Freud upon sociology in the United States. *American Journal of Psychiatry,* 45(3), 356–374.

Burnham, J. C. (1960). Psychiatry, psychology and the regressive movement. *American Quarterly,* 12, 457–465.

Davis, A. and Dollard, J. (1940). *Children of bondage.* Washington, DC: American Council on Education.

Dollard, J. (1935). *Criteria for the life history: With analysis of six notable documents.* New York: Peter Smith.

Dollard, J. (1937). *Caste and class in a southern town.* New York: Harper and Brothers.

Fancher, R. E. (1973). *Psychiatric psychology: The development of Freud's thought.* New York: W. W. Norton.

Friedman, L. J. (2013). *The lives of Erich Fromm: Love's prophet.* New York: Columbia University Press.

Frosh, S. (2013). Psychoanalysis, colonialism, racism. *Journal of Theoretical and Philosophical Psychology,* 33, 141–154.

Gilman, S. L. (1985). *Difference and pathology: Stereotypes of sexuality, race, and madness.* Ithaca: Cornell University Press.

Grob, G. N. (1983). *Mental illness and American society,* 1875–1940. Princeton: Princeton University Press.

Hale Jr., N. G. (1995). *The rise and crisis of psychoanalysis in the United States: Freud and the Americans*, 1917–1985. New York: Oxford University Press.

Haller Jr., J. (1994). *Medical protestants: The eclectics in American medicine*, 1925–1939. Carbondale, IL: Southern Illinois University Press.

Johnson, C. (1952). Sullivan's contribution to sociology. In Mullahy, P. (Ed.), *The contributions of Harry Stack Sullivan: A symposium on interpersonal theory in psychiatry and social sciences*. New York: Hermitage House.

Johnson, C. S. (1938–1940). Correspondence between Charles S. Johnson and Harry S. Sullivan. In *Records of the Institute of Human Relations*. Folder 134, Box 13, 1938–1940, Special Collections/Archives, John Hope and Aurelia E. Franklin Library. Nashville, TN: Fisk University.

Kluckhohn, F. R. (1940). The participant-observer technique in small communities. *American Journal of Sociology*, 46, 331–343.

Lasswell, H. (1928). Papers, Folders 782 and 783, Box *56, 1928, Manuscript and Archives*. New Haven, CT: Yale University Library.

Lasswell, H. (1930/1977). *Psychopathology and politics*. Chicago, IL: University of Chicago Press.

Lunbeck, E. (1994). *The psychiatric persuasion: Knowledge, gender, and power in modern America*. Princeton, NJ: Princeton University Press.

Manson, W. C. (1988). *The psychodynamics of culture: Abram Kardiner and neo-Freudian anthropology*. New York: Greenwood Press.

Mayo, E. (1937). Psychiatry and sociology in relation to social disorganization. *American Journal of Sociology*, 42, 825–831.

Mead, M. (1932). *The changing culture of an Indian tribe*. New York: Columbia University Press.

Mead, M. (1935) More comprehensive field methods. *American Anthropologist*, 35, 1–15.

Perry, H. S. (1972). Sapir, Jean and Philip (interview with Jean Sapir, the wife of Edward Sapir, August 17, 1972. *Helen Swick Perry papers*. In possession of Stuart Perry. Cambridge, MA.

Perry, H. S. (1982). *Psychiatrist of America: The life of Harry Stack Sullivan*. Cambridge, MA: Harvard University Press.

Rose, A. C. (2005). Putting the South on the psychological map: The impact of region and race on the human sciences in the 1930s. *The Journal of Southern History*, 71, 321–356.

Rothstein, W. (1987). *American medical schools and the practice of medicine: A history*. New York: Oxford University Press.

Sapir, E. (1937). The contribution of psychiatry to and understanding of behavior in society. *American Journal of Sociology*, 42, 862–870.

Sargent, S. S. and Smith, M. W. (Eds.). (1949). *Culture and personality*. New York, NY: Viking Fund.

Stanton, A. and Schwartz, S. (1954). *The mental hospital: A study of institutional participation in psychiatric illness and treatment.* New York, NY: Basic Books.

Sullivan, H. S. (1926, circa). *Projected book: Psychopathology of youth.* Washington, DC: Washington School of Psychiatry Archive.

Sullivan, H. S. (1929a). *Schizophrenia as a human process.* New York: Norton.

Sullivan, H. S. (1929b). Discussion of Lawson G. Lowrey, "The study of personality." *American Journal of Psychiatry,* 86, 700–702.

Sullivan, H. S. (1931). Training of the general medical student in psychiatry. *American Journal of Orthopsychiatry,* 1, 371–379.

Sullivan, H. S. (1934). Discussion of Erich Lindemann and William Malamud, "Experimental analysis of the psychopathological effects of intoxicating drugs," *American Journal of Psychiatry,* 90, 879–881.

Sullivan, H. S. (1938a). Editorial note: The William Alanson White Psychiatric Foundation. *Psychiatry,* 1, 135–140.

Sullivan, H. S. (1938b). Editorial note: The William Allison White Psychiatric Foundation. *Psychiatry,* 1, 140–141.

Sullivan, H. S. (1939). The support of psychiatric research and training. *Psychiatry,* 2, 273–297.

Sullivan, H. S. (1940). Discussion of the case of Warren Wall. In Frazier, E. F. (Ed.), *Negro youth at the crossways: Their personality development in the middle states* (pp. 228–234). Washington, DC: American Council of Education.

Sullivan, H. S. (1941). Memorandum on a psychiatric reconnaissance. In Johnson, C. S. (Ed.), *Growing up in the black belt: Negro youth in the rural south* (pp. 328–333). Washington, DC: American Council of Education.

Sullivan, H. S. (1947). Ten years of *Psychiatry*: A statement by the editor. *Psychiatry,* 10, 433–435.

Sullivan, H. S. (1972). *Personal psychopathology: Early formulations.* New York: Norton.

Thompson, C. and Mullahy, P. (1950). *Psychoanalysis: Evolution and development.* New York: Hermitage House.

William Alanson White Psychiatric Foundation. (1939). Bulletin: Washington School of Psychiatry. *Psychiatry,* 2, 473(I)–477(V).

Williams, F. (1928) Psychiatry and its relation to the teaching of medicine. *American Journal of Psychiatry,* 85, 689–700.

Chapter 2

Anthropology and Psychoanalysis
A Lost Dialogue Over Time

Victoria Malkin

In 1909, Sigmund Fre ud travelled to Clark University for a conference to introduce psychoanalysis to the United States, at the invitation of its president G. Stanley Hall, renowned psychologist and the
first president of the American Psychological Association. Franz
Boas (1858–1942), the father of American anthropology and preem-
inent scholar of the time, was also there. Boas had been invited to
give his paper on "Psychological Problems of Anthropology." His talk
advocated that anthropology should look for universal laws of human
psychological functioning, but only through the use of detailed ethnography and analysis of unique cultural contexts (Groark, 2019).
This initial encounter between the two towering figures of psychoanalysis and anthropology ended with their divergence that continues
to this day, and here I explore some of these encounters and separa-
tions to this present day. Why, we might ask, would two fields both
devoted to an understanding of human experience in all its particularity end up virtually ignoring what each might offer to the other?
How did Boas' culture have so little to do with Freud's civilization,
even though both men shared a belief in the role of empirical observation alongside enlightenment ideals? Both fields were born within
the contours of 19th century thought and its desire to think about
the human, a liberal ideal, who could be understood and represented
through science. Both fields asked us to be observers of ourselves.
Our observing ego was to be put to use to understand the individual
or culture – a position that both psychoanalysis and anthropology
have come to critique. Yet, even with this shared critique, neither
finds any solace in their current position as outsiders pleading for

DOI: 10.4324/9781003270355-3

complexity in a world that looks for reductive understanding. This chapter begins with this first encounter, then takes up some of the strands of anthropological thinking that remained known and not known, repressed and ignored within the psychoanalytic mainstream, even within the interpersonal tradition that in its early iteration seriously attempted a dialogue with some of the most influential anthropologists in that time.

At this groundbreaking conference, Boas' plea was for a particularism that could, he hoped, lead to the universal. Boas was in fact arguing against the popular ideas of cultural evolution that animated the 19th century "armchair" anthropologists who catalogued cultures into areas and races, and then subsequently classified "primitive" cultures as a stand-in for an earlier stage in human history. With this freezing of so-called primitive cultures into an evolutionary timeline, their rituals, religions, kinship systems and political arrangements were placed on the early end of this timeline, which landed at the door of the 19th century gentleman of European civilization.

In contrast to Boas, Freud's paper launched his new method and theory of the human psyche. Freud presented on the opening day, after Clark asked Boas to cede his time to later in the program so as to welcome the European guest. Freud's burgeoning interest and writings using evolutionary anthropology blossomed after this conference, alongside his liberal use of its ethnographic data to validate and inspire his more esoteric ideas. While there is no official record that Freud attended Boas' talk, from his blossoming interest in evolutionary anthropological ideas after the meeting, it is thought that not only was he most likely there, but that Boas' plea fell on deaf ears as Freud took up the very evolutionary model that Boas was critiquing (Kenny, 2015). Boas was moving away from a unilineal theory of cultural evolution while Freud actively embraced it. Freud would successively elaborate on a theory of culture, leading him to conclude that the human psyche contained the traces of human origins where history and myth would meet. He would continue to elaborate a sweeping model of human history based on drives and mythic murders and held on to a developmental model of cultural evolution in order to bolster his emerging ideas developed later in *Totem and Taboo* – a book where Freud located remnants of human history in the psyche itself. For Freud, human culture and history was now encoded into our very psychological structure.

Boas in the meantime would spend his life publishing detailed analyses of specific cultures and histories to uncover meanings within their particular systems (cf. King, 2019). Boas used ethnographic data to reject the eugenic positions of earlier evolutionary theories which saw primitive cultures as coterminous with early humans. In this 19th century thought, European man had travelled further on the long and arduous journey towards his enlightenment, while primitive man remained at the back of the line. Evolutionary theory posited that the culture of the primitive was transformed into the civilization of the European over time, a high culture that was entwined with rationality which was achieved only after passing through previous cultural stages. In this conceptualization of culture, there was no need to study primitive culture in context, because culture was already mapped onto an evolutionary structure that was predetermined.

Freud's ongoing excavations into this earlier anthropological literature, such as James Frazer and Edward Tylor in the UK or Lewis Henry Morgan in the US, ignored the detailed work by Boas on native American Culture, as well as his later work with the children of recent immigrants in the US (Pierpoint, 2004). For Freud, ethnology was there to generate theories of a psyche that reflected our ontogenic beginnings. Not only was primitive man, this cultural Other, equated with a historical stage in man's evolutionary history, it was now also an Other fixated, or stuck, in a psychoneurotic stage akin to a child. In other words, Freud inscribed evolution into psychic life; primitives and children were locked into the same playpen. Historical time and psychosexual stages were interchangeable. The primitive, a criminal in the making, was now arrested and locked out of history, forever stuck in mythic time, dependent on magical thinking, murderous feelings and barred from the rationality and higher thinking of the European ego. Primitive man was enveloped in his primitive defenses: the savage with his primary process who remained hostage to the pleasure principal and dependent on his totem and omnipotent Gods, unable to escape. Law and morals, superego and reality principle were part of civilization, something the savage lacked. The savage luxuriated in his dream life and myth, the European developed his ego and sublimation.

Boas and Freud, along with G. Stanley Hall[1], could thus be seen as akin to transitional objects, moving 19th century thought into a 20th century modernism, but never quite removing its traces. They put forward universal theories that could encompass culture and psychology as they aspired to uncover some basic structures of human experience. But Freud and Hall (and Boas to a lesser extent) could never quite shake off the Victorian morality plays, remaining trapped in their local cultural ideologies, even though Freud offered his own radical break and revolutionary ideas for his time. Both revolutionary in their ideas, Boas and Freud resisted any mutual influence, refusing to absorb the others' ideas into their developing inquiries. They rejected the implications of each other's mode of thought and repressed the challenge each theory might have on their intellectual labor. Boas would not entertain the idea of an unconscious that might determine aspects of culture and Freud was rarely interested in the specificity of cultural forms and their meanings outside of a circular logic where denial becomes proof. A putative dialogue between the disciplines remained oppositional rather than collaborative. Each discipline became a mirror to the other, shedding light on what has been left out and confirming the failure of any one theory to complete a narrative of human subjectivity.

In spite of their differences, anthropology and psychoanalysis both represented enlightenment attempts to search for master narratives of human experience. Both modes of thinking shared a desire to find the underpinning and laws of human functioning. Psychoanalysis laid out deliberations on libido theory and a fundamental (Oedipal) law that organized social lives. This was in fact taken up by some anthropologists, both in Europe and in the United States, who searched for an Oedipal structure using ethnographic data within different kinship systems. [2] They asked, in essence, where and how nature transformed into culture and where the boundary between these two forces lay. The transition for Freud was conflict driven, a grand bargain that entailed loss of one pleasure in exchange for another: the pleasure of being part of civilization. This melancholic pleasure remained full of desire for the lost Other that remained closer to nature – coded as those primitive others admired and reviled for their existence in nature. Meanwhile for the anthropologist, culture was the mechanism that enabled the transmission of something human, something beyond nature. If the anthropologists marked the 'primitive' as closer to nature, that did not leave him or her further from culture, it just helped mark a contrast.

Boas and his students painstakingly documented how cultural traits were context dependent, showing how similar behaviors and beliefs could serve completely different functions and meanings. Anthropology was finding different complex systems of kinships and laws that generated social life and power in specific cultural contexts. For Freud, a Totem was always a Totem – a structure in the unconscious – while for Boas, its meanings were multiple and represented complex local and migratory histories and cosmologies. Whereas Freud saw a representation of underlying psychic structure inherited via a Lamarkian theory of inheritance, Boas saw history and culture. Where Freud saw obsessive rituals and magical thinking underlying neurotics and religious belief, Boas saw symbolic meaning, ritual transformation and values and norms. Boas believed that Freud had taken anthropological data and resorted to fanciful ideas with little scientific evidence. As Boas' student, Alexander Goldenweiser, summarized in 1922,

> The assumption of a psychic continuity between the generations is but an alluring fantasy and the willingness to accept it as true, in the face of contradictory historic and biologic evidence, may well be regarded as a curious example of that omnipotence of thought which Freud regards as characteristic of the psychic life of primitive man and of the neurotic.
>
> (cited in Groark, 2019, p. 565)

Freud left texts and works that have enabled multiple readings, embedded with the possibility of reworking and rethinking the ways in which humans remain unknown to themselves. But ultimately, Freud's own desire for psychoanalysis to be understood as a science, a narrative that could rise above others, blinded him to what in the end, one might say, was another corner of the scientific avant-garde of the time. While Boas was struggling for a theory that would validate and pay homage to difference, challenging eugenic and racist theories of the day, Freud would cling to a desire for an account of psychic life that would place human diversity within mythic structures, ironically erasing historical particularity for the group, while advocating fiercely for its place within the individual. Culture was less relevant; what mattered was the individual's epic struggle to survive it. The insertion of a mythic structure now lodged in the unconscious leaves Freud as the master in his own house, father of the psychoanalytic movement where "psychoanalysis, is always, without question, is [my] work alone" (Freud, 1914, p. 8). Culture, that topic that fueled anthropology, was rendered mute as the science of subjectivity rose from its ashes.

Anthropological Confrontations with Psychological Models

The 1938 articles in *Psychiatry* by Edward Sapir (1884–1939) and Ruth Benedict (1887–1948) both represent the emergent second generation of Boasian anthropologists. This generation embraced an idea of culture as formative to a group, just as their teacher had, but they further elaborated on the interrelation of psychology and culture. Their research led them to scrutinize their own culture, albeit still with certain inherent biases. They were no longer solely the objective observers of a distant Other as they moved to critique norms and traits closer to home. They exchanged (Freudian) civilization for a kaleidoscope of cultures and highlighted the importance of specific sets of shared understandings. Culture for these Boasians enabled the shorthand necessary for what Harry Stack Sullivan would call consensual validation. A validation based on a desire for understanding within interpersonal relations, as opposed to misunderstanding and misrecognition. And a consensus only thinkable if that desire resides within a fantasy of understanding that is enabled by the context of a shared culture.

Taken together, these articles begin to question how and where we might locate the difference produced through culture. Would we find *"Patterns of Culture"* that transcend and organize human difference, as proposed by Benedict (1934) in her well-known book of that name? Or following Sapir, is it the case that culture is an abstraction conceptualized for social scientists who locate difference back onto the individual? For Benedict and Sapir alike, child development was implicit in the way in which culture created difference (Benedict) and in the process by which culture became internalized and individualized (Sapir). Their explorations remain contemporary in their concern. The quest for something that makes us all *human*, whether rooted in biology, culture or Freud's mythic unconscious, continues within the social sciences today. We appear to be fueled by our desperate desire to find that something that can be deemed precultural and presocial and that would satisfy our anxiety that there must be more than a perpetual difference. Yet we end up most usually with a universalism that reifies western ideals around self, humans, bodies and experiences that are imbued with specific notions of what it is to be a person in a particular (western industrialized) space.

The Boasian lineage of anthropologists was focused on heterogeneity between cultures. Released from the Victorian diorama of the civilizations of man, cultures were now compared and elaborated in terms of their own sets of internal patterns and meanings. Both Sapir (fig 2) and Benedict (fig 3) saw culture as framing and organizing our most intimate life and interactions. Its invisibility for the participant was the result of its internalization, not due to its absence. For Sapir, culture was the unconscious patterns that shape life. Sapir's origin as a talented linguist of Native American languages led him to value an unconscious form, which he saw as akin to the underlying form of a language – the encompassing form that permits the specificity of rules and grammar (Irvine, 2002). In our mother tongue, we instantly recognize grammar mistakes, but the form that contains and organizes them remain out of our awareness. Form is rendered visible when it encounters difference – as Sapir would show for both language and culture (Sapir, 2002a). We are most aware of our culture when we are removed from it. It looms when absent, coming into sharp relief when one is othered to the extent that commonsensical ideas are put at risk, and incommensurable difference can shatter dialogue.

If Sapir was interested in the mechanisms that wound language and culture together, Benedict's book, *Patterns of Culture* (1934) took a broader view, comparing three cultures to investigate how culture organizes social life. For Benedict, any given culture was one example within a vast array of possibilities. Cultures were differently integrated wholes which set limits on what was possible for those who lived within

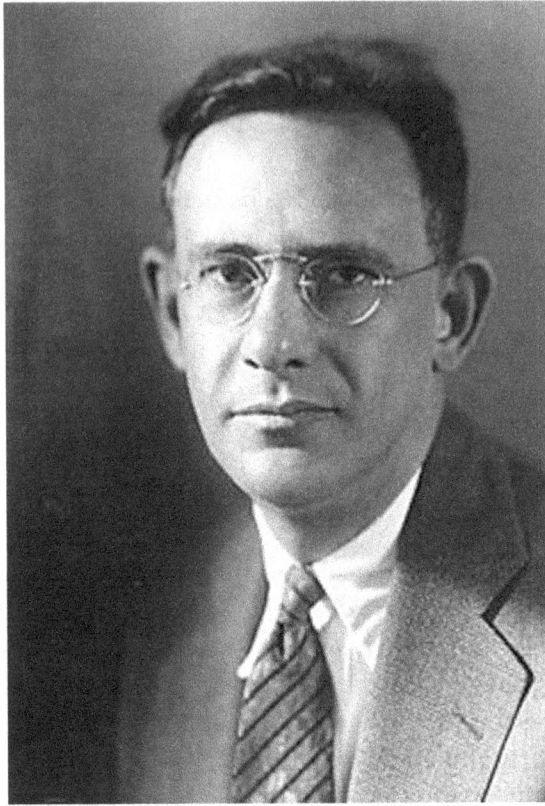

Figure 2 Edward Sapir, Historic Images/Alamy Stock Photo.

them. Benedict, the originator of the term cultural relativity, challenged the moralism of her times. She contemplated what patterns she could find, coming up with the concept of Apollonian and Dionysian practices that define different cultures. She began with social practices emergent in the earliest part of the lifecycle through to its end and explored how these practices consolidated ideals and meaning for those within it. "A culture, like an individual," to quote Benedict, "is a more or less a consistent pattern of thought and action" (1934, p. 46), and thus emerged a loosely assorted group of scholars known as the Culture and Personality school in anthropology. While this group was ultimately faulted for creating a deterministic and reductionist version of the person in culture, Benedict and her circle were responding to their intuition that culture generated radical difference, without

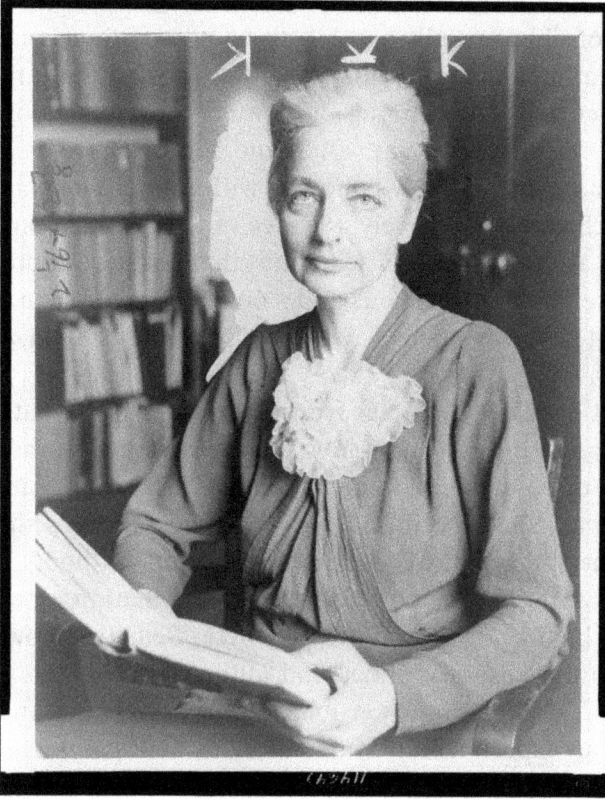

Figure 3 Ruth Benedict, 1937, Library of Congress.

placing this within prior hierarchical thinking of previous anthropologists (LeVine, 2002).

Benedict's 1938 article, *Continuity and Discontinuity in Cultural Conditioning*, is considered one of her classics in anthropology, and introduces us to how persuasive Benedict was in her elaboration of cultural ideals and conflicts. She uses a comparative method to show how varied social organization can be and, in turn, forces us to interrogate our own beliefs. Benedict begins with what she argues is a universal transition from the child (son) to the adult (father). What might appear to be an inevitable fact of nature, she states, is as much a social achievement as a natural life cycle development. It is, she says, a transition that has been universalized from our own cultural vantage point. Benedict takes the binaries that she proposes as the natural arc from son to father – submission to dominance, irresponsible to responsible, sexually naïve to sexually active and considers how different cultures organize this transition in ways that are (dis)continuous over time. In outlining the conflicts engendered by the transition as a question of social values and conflicting roles, the article foreshadows contemporary concerns within interpersonal and relational psychoanalysis, namely, the idea of the dissociation of human capacities: affects, ideas and self-states that coalesce in order to sustain interpersonal interactions and a coherent self-system. Sullivan's *not-me* that hovers outside of awareness so as to sustain a *me* in interaction with you.

Benedict provides examples from a wide range of what she terms continuous cultures to show how child rearing, alongside cultural ideologies of what a child can do, enable a smooth journey from son to father. She describes accepted social practices that forge a path for the child to move towards his role in adulthood; a tide that moves the child gently towards his new destination as opposed to a chasm which he must jump to get there. Benedict shows cultures that encourage responsibilities and autonomy from young ages so that the transition to a responsible adult is continuous and gradual, alongside an experimentation that enables multiple social positions of reciprocity and kinship relationships and which locate the child in and out of submissive and dominant positions, among others, thus preparing them for adult roles. Finally, she highlights the children's exposure to sexual play and sexuality in a manner that neither assumes innocence nor pathologizes childhood sexuality. In continuous cultures, argues Benedict, the child is not dropped into his new paternal role unprepared for its script. In comparison, discontinuous cultures contain stark differences between expectations in different life stages. However, as Benedict briefly describes, most discontinuous cultures resolve this conflict through the introduction of ritual practices and initiations that move cohorts through age grades to guide their transitions and mark their entry into a new subject position alongside peers.

After all this, the article in fact reveals Benedict in the final page; there, in a crescendo that returns her home, she questions the universal psychological stages that were at the heart of psychology (and psychoanalysis) during her era. In the final paragraph, she aims her arrow, confronting the popular idea of adolescence which had in fact been theorized by G. Stanley Hall (2004), the psychologist at the heart of the Freud and Boas encounter. At the turn of the century, Hall had theorized adolescence as a necessary and universal period of conflict, a *Strurm and Drang*, brought on by the child's life cycle changes, but which Benedict now reconceptualizes as a cultural conflict. For Benedict, western culture had reneged on those cultural ideologies and practices that could support the demands of puberty, abandoning the child to adolescence and a confrontation with a mutinous body, while simultaneously lacking any ritual practices or cultural ideologies that could support him or her, such as those she had observed elsewhere. In contrast to Hall, she concludes the "problem" of adolescence is neither a biological certainty nor an individual conflict, but a cultural problem that had been rebranded as a psychological one and relocated as a problem of the individual. As Benedict writes, "we invoke a physiological scheme to account for neurotic adjustments (and) we are led to overlook the possibility of developing social institutions which would lessen the social cost we now pay; instead we elaborate a set of dogmas which prove inapplicable under other social conditions" (1938, p. 167).

Benedict opens our eyes to the cultural repertoires available to organize life, and with this, puts in question our own ethnocentric versions of psychology and development, a problem that continues to this day as universal assumptions about development are assumed, based on research that takes place chiefly in WEIRD societies (western, educated, industrialized, rich and democratic), and most normally among the subset of the white middle class (Lancy, 2008). For Benedict and Margaret Mead, both Boas' students and sporadic lovers, their intimacy and non-conformist sexuality and gender roles gave them a window from which to challenge their own culture. At the same time, their research exploring other societies elsewhere was part of their struggle to account for their own sense of alienation (King, 2019). While their ethnographies can walk the tightrope between exotification and generalizations, their attempts to open a space for a discussion of gender roles, childhood sexuality and variation was unique in their era. Margaret Mead would later move to critique the psychoanalytic idea of neurotic fixations at oral, anal and genital stages based on Freud's version of child development with her use of ethnographic content to address various childhood developmental stages she rebranded as lap, knee and yard babies that were developmental transitions determined as much by culture as the developmental map of erogenous zones alone (Mead, 2008). Both women challenged the prurient sexuality of their day as well as its 19th century racialized stereotypes. Had they been taken seriously by the psychoanalytic establishment of their time, perhaps they could have created a diversion away from the more normative ideology that American psychoanalysis embraced in the 1950s, with its focus on adaptation and its reliance on ego psychology.

Following a short affair with Margaret Mead, Sapir was never quite as comfortable confronting the sexual mores of his day. But in contrast to Benedict, Sapir speaks to contemporary anthropological and psychoanalytic concerns around the questions of individual agency and its limits within culture. While Benedict took a bird's eye view of a particular culture and its ideals, Sapir began from the ground up. His writings cut a trajectory from a brilliant linguist to a theorist who would engage the theme of psychology and culture through the question of the individual. Sapir's 1938 article "Why Cultural Anthropology Needs the Psychiatrist," is one of his last. It was written at a time when he was critiquing anthropologists for what he felt were their crass generalizations and easy psychologizing of cultures – something Sapir called the "as if" psychology of culture (Sapir, 2002b). While not naming Benedict, he was a frequent objector to broad generalizations that named cultures as paranoid, obsessive or hysterical (Sapir, 1934). As a linguist, Sapir had spent time not only classifying numerous native American and first nation languages, but he also ascribed to the Boasian idea that language could only be studied and understood by its usage in context and explained through its own terms as if being represented by a native user. He maintained a structural view that language forms remained embedded in the unconscious, creating unconscious patterning, but he fiercely prized the possibility of self-expression within this.[3]

Towards the end of his life, Sapir was suspicious of any idea of culture that painted it in the abstract. He challenged social scientists and anthropologists who located culture on a metaphysical plane and argued instead that culture is in reality present, lived and reproduced through individuals. In his 1938 article, Sapir demonstrates this problem from the question of epistemology: that is, how one can come to know and claim knowledge of a given culture. From where does one derive this authority to knowledge claims? Sapir exposes the mystification that enables cultural analysis, reminding us that this always and only emerges through interpretations of information gathered from and through an Other. His article illustrates by examining the text of a well-known book by the ethnologist J.O. Dorsey on *Omaha Sociology*. The author, unusually for the times, introduced casual acknowledgements of discord among his informants who disagreed about cultural explanations, statements which Sapir summarizes as *"Two Crows denies this."* In these sparks of singularity and disagreement, Sapir begins to elaborate his complex theory of culture and the individual. Sapir observes that there will necessarily be divergent lives and interpretations of a culture from those who live within it.

Sapir was convinced that detailed observations of interpersonal relations – the place where culture was located and produced – were needed. According to Sapir, in his refusal, Two Crows was neither necessarily outside culture, psychotic, nor wrong in his denial. There might be myriads of reasons for Two Crows's denial. And even if he was psychotic, his stance might be on the cusp of initiating a revolution which could bring people into a new understanding and would initiate a new tradition over time. For Sapir, culture and tradition are expressed and made through interactions. There is no consensus that can describe culture, even though its unconscious patterning may provide certain forms. Sapir takes us directly into the realm of the interpersonal and language where, according to him, symbols are always personal and cultural: "One suspects that the symbolic role of words has an importance for the solution of our problems. after all if A calls B a liar he creates a reverberating cosmos of potential action and judgement. And the fatal word can be passed on to C, the society and culture is complete" (Sapir, 1937, p. 870).

In making this claim, Sapir and Freudian versions of psychoanalysis are more in agreement then he might care to acknowledge. Sapir locates culture in this triangulation of meaning, perhaps akin to the Freudian Oedipal position which for Freud was when culture emerges in a super-ego (or as Lacan would later suggest, where the subject is ushered into the symbolic via the paternal signifier – language – and without which remains locked in an imaginary world of the mirror stage). Sapir, however, was more interested in the dilemma of how to separate out something called culture from the individual. He further questions the conceptual distinction between culture and personality. For the child, he argues, all learning and discovery of the world could be called cultural learning; a learning that allows the child to be in a specific world. And yet over time, this is transformed for the individual into something akin to personality in the adult. He concludes that these concepts are impossible to separate: one can neither assert a general culture that would encompass the individuals who live within it, nor assume a personality that emerges within a culture. For Sapir, the separate realms of culture and personality are merely heuristic. They serve as markers, or ideas, that permit us to navigate our experience of the world and the other. The distinction allows for "intelligent and helpful growth because each is based on a distinctive type of imaginative participation by the observer in the life around him" (Sapir, 1934, p. 409). Furthermore, Sapir warns of the reductive danger when thinking about culture, especially for those who are radically different and remain a cultural other, whose individuality is so easily erased in broad brushstrokes. Taking on his peers and with a nod to Freud, he cautions:

> It seems unexpectedly difficult to conjure up the image of live people in intelligibly live relationships in those areas defined as primitive. The personalities that inhabit our ethnological monographs seem almost schizoid in their unemotional acceptance of the heavy colors, tapestries, and furniture of their ethnological stage. Is it any wonder that actors so vaguely conceived... can be bludgeoned by a more persistent intelligence than theirs into sawing wood for still remoter stages, say that dread drama of the slain father and the birth of totemism?
>
> (Sapir, 1937, p. 865)

Sapir foreshadows debates that would take hold much later, not only in his critique of culture and its metaphysical location, but with his focus on the individual, agency and imagination within the confines of form. Sapir's ideas in many ways prove the more enduring over time with his inquiry centered on the ways that people use their symbolic worlds to fashion themselves as singular beings. In contrast, the Culture and Personality movement disbanded in spite of it having been the most notorious and bestselling corner of anthropological thinking to date. Over time, it became a caricature of itself as it attempted to integrate psychoanalytic ideas about early childcare practices as determinative of cultural models and ideals. Nevertheless, to discount its thinking is to ignore how Benedict and her colleagues, with their descriptions of culture and their portraits of difference, still resonate. Their desire to humanize the Other and perhaps more importantly, their attempt to open a space to difference, was a disruption that could ultimately cast doubt on ourselves.

From the Psychological Self to the Subject of Culture

Benedict and Sapir precede the current era in anthropology where questions of power and representation have become central, alongside a steady critique of the notion that culture is a closed homogenous system of values and practices. Nevertheless, they initiated questions that continue today. Their writing opens a window into the earlier anthropologists who attempted to theorize the problem of cultural difference – with questions around how to conceptualize its origins, how to think about where it resides, and how to represent it. In fact, culture as an organizing principle has moved into the background in anthropology, exchanged for debates around individual agency and social change. The question of the culture and psyche has itself shifted towards the idea that the self is as much culturally determined as a type of universal agency. The Subject is produced through culture as opposed to standing outside of it. Meanwhile in psychoanalysis, the failure to address a theory of culture becomes more urgent as culture itself moves so rapidly, generating new and different subjects in the consulting room.

The 1938 articles of Benedict and Sapir also foreshadow contemporary psychoanalytic discussions where the question of culture looms large, but with no coherent agreement of how to theorize it or its manifestation within the clinical dyad. With movements from the idea of the social unconscious (Layton, 2006), to those who use the Critical Theory of the Frankfurt School to think of us as subjects who are interpellated by the Other of culture (Dimen, 2011), to Culture as a self-Object (Peters, 2010) or to how cultural norms influence counter-transference and normative views of subject making (Bonovitz, 2005; Fisek, 2010; Reiss, 2005), psychoanalytic writing seems to posit culture as anything and everything. In spite of the attention to culture in the Interpersonal and Relational school, there is little consensus on its impact on the subject or its influence in the room. The limits of its importance seem arbitrary in most treatments and idiosyncratic to the clinician. In our clinics, we are more aware than ever that we can never be outside of culture and ideally alert to the normativity that can pervade our formulations, aware how easy it is to pathologize the other as Benedict argued (1938). And yet as psychoanalysts, we struggle with the paradox that while interpersonal interactions (clinical or other) are the locus and production of culture as Sapir would argue, we lack the theoretical tools that would formulate this. There is little sense of how to assess what impact culture has within the moment to moment inquiry into our dyadic explosions of misunderstandings. There is neither a question on the role of culture in the formation of a symptom (Benedict), nor, returning to Sapir, exploration of how the line between culture and personality is itself more heuristic than absolute, leaving the clinician with few guidelines as to where the line might be drawn.

After having studied anthropology, I began my psychoanalytic training in the mid 2000's; in retrospect, I began with minimal exposure to psychoanalysis, most of it via the poststructuralist and feminist schools in anthropology that were current at the time. Anthropology had redirected debates over "Culture," abandoning the more collective Durkheimian version of a community that had led to an overemphasis on collective representations and their power to subsume the individual. The idealized homogenous community was deconstructed and shown to be a denial of the complex reality of the Other. A critique was developed of the binary where literate cultures were given history while oral cultures were locked into myth. Anthropology was forced into its own reckoning; its history and constitution as a discipline exposed as intrinsic to the very creation of the concept of culture that was a strait jacket for those it described, a fantasy of the anthropologist more than a concept that could represent the lives of others. The (de)construction of the Other and culture became inherent to the discipline and its teaching (Moore ,2007). By the early 90's, anthro-pology was less focused on culture as a variable of analysis, ironically clearing the room just in time for the army of cultural competency and diversity trainings to break down the doors stomping over the major critiques of the concept of culture that anthropology had elaborated over the decades.

Anthropology had shifted – more intent on showing how, in col-lectively orientated societies as much as in our own individualized ones, the psyche was never completely captured by culture, as had been crudely represented by some of the worst of the culture and personality school. Theories now moved to decentering the subject and looking at the ways in which agency was circumscribed within differential power relations. Some schools of anthropology rejected any association with psychology as relevant to cultural analysis. For example, Clifford Geertz argued that the description of culture – its webs of significance and meaning – were a separate province and reg-ister from personal psychology (cf. LeVine, 2014). Others, especially those working on questions of gender, race and colonialization, would advocate for the unconscious as the force that freed the subject from discourse. They theorized and looked for agency outside of hegem-ony, both at the level of the individual and then to think about how change takes place. For this group, Lacan, and the symbolic of cul-ture became important in that it located the external culture along-side the question of the imaginary, or imagination, to be an engine of social change. The question of deep motivation, and whether this had to be understood within the Oedipal parameters or something else, remains a larger unresolved debate (Moore, 2007).

The dialogue that had been tenuously initiated between anthro-pology and psychoanalysis remained more than ever at the margins. For psychoanalysis in the US, with the rise of the ego psychologists, with their focus on ego and adaptation, culture became something external. It was perceived as a problem because of its pressure on the drives, but irrelevant to internal life. At the same time, culture was also being read as a text and interpreted as a product of drive derivatives, an expression of infantile wishes, conflicts or sublima-tion. Thus, paradoxically, culture could be both the cause of repres-sion while also simultaneously being its end point. Meanwhile, in the cultural school of psychoanalysis, which would later became known as the Interpersonal school (Frie, 2014), culture was taken seriously as both external and causal, but mostly to challenge the drive theory of the Freudians. It could produce certain neuroses or personalities, as elaborated in the works of Erich Fromm (1944), Karen Horney (1937) or Alfred Kardiner (Stocking, 1986a) – but no clear theory or meta-psychology was agreed upon to organize the relationship of culture to psyche (Molino, 2004). Sullivan's ideas about parataxic distortions and the not-me that emerges in the context of interpersonal interactions suggest that the importance of context and language use is key to many of his diagnostic observations. But Sullivan suggests little in the way of a roadmap to consider the role of culture outside of individual misunderstandings between people that cause the self system to adapt (and in this one sees the influence of Sapir).

During my training, there was little exploration of culture – by then the one class devoted to it was primarily focused on questions of race and counter-transference – in spite of the role of culture in the history of the interpersonal school. Not that it was not held as important, but there was little in the way of discussions of what that importance was. Culture was in essence reduced to the role of external reality or context. The question of the complicated relationship between culture and psyche as begun by Sapir and Benedict and taken up by Sullivan or Fromm was generally simplified to the question of internal versus external reality, to the real mother as opposed to the fantasied mother, the real family as opposed to the Oedipal fantasy, and trauma as produced by events as opposed to fantasy. In spite of Fromm's work, which in some ways parallels the Culture and Personality movement in its analysis of authoritarianism and capitalism as values and ideals that produce certain ways of being in the world, and Sullivan's pioneering work on Schizophrenia as the product of disordered social relations, alongside his focus on the peer group as core to the development of the person as separate from the family (Hegarty, 2005), there was no attempt to integrate these questions into a revisionist history of Interpersonal Psychoanalysis. To this day, while there is a growing literature on race and power, mostly at the edges of the discipline, but now galloping towards the center due to current events, there remains little sense of what if anything we might understand culture to be – or how to consider the same questions that were outlined by Sapir and Benedict years ago.

The drawbridge between anthropology and psychoanalysis seems to have firmly shut, even though psychoanalysis is currently confronted with the question of cultural difference more than ever. Moreover, there are multiple strands of research within anthropology that might prove disruptive to some of the more normative models in psychoanalytic thinking, especially those that arrived via psychology and psychiatry. Research on childhood development, an area Sapir himself felt would reveal much about the relationship between culture and psychology (2002b, p. 197), highlights the vast repertoire of child development models that point to the difficulty of ascribing any sort of presocial beginnings. Winnicott's baby is not just dependent on a mother but constituted within a culture. Even in the first 12 months, the vast arena of accepted childcare models, along with ideas about what a baby is and what they need, have a cultural repertoire that challenge western childcare models. Suzanne Gaskins (2006) has shown how modes of communication and interaction vary from birth in ways that have outcomes to personhood. Meanwhile, biological anthropology clearly verifies the basic needs of the child for ongoing non-disruptive attachments. But ethnographic data finds variation in how that plays out and what it looks like in different settings, finding that even in hunter gather tribes who share the most similar ecological niches and demands, (cultural) variation is documented in weaning and childcare models (Konner, 2016). The idea of mirroring attunement and facial responsiveness as encouraged by Beebe, for example, has little predictive value with Innuit children who spend their early life on their mothers' backs looking out at the world (Briggs, 1970) or Beng babies who are passed around and appreciated in large circles from birth and as a result are found to have less stranger anxiety (Gottlieb, 2004), or finally German children, who were more likely to be classified as avoidant attachment, because self sufficiency was valued from an early age (LeVine and Norman, 2008).

Attachment theory has emerged as one of the more contemporary developmental models for psychoanalytic theorizing among the relational and interpersonal schools, where its styles are essentially mapped onto a dissociative model, or some sort of internalized object relations, with self-states or not-me moments representing attachment disorders as the individual struggles with ambivalence and safety. Nevertheless, there is no appreciation of the ways that attachment styles as elaborated by psychology perpetuates certain American middle-class ideals of childhood and relationships which may pathologize those who developed elsewhere. The model itself, with its focus on a certain type of expressive emotional closeness, holds a mirror onto the white middle class, frustrating many of those whose lives cannot live up to this cultural model (Quinn, 2013; Mageo, 2013). On top of this, ideas of agency, which are perpetuated in American childcare from birth on, where in-comprehending babies are offered choices from birth by loving parents and are congratulated when the right choice is made are in themselves reiterations of individualized models of (self-governing) selves brought up within nuclear families (Gaskins, 2006).

From a position outside of the basic research that might place some of our psychoanalytic or psychological models at risk, perhaps even more disruptive for us is the problem of how psychoanalytic discourse is part of the constitution of what we observe. The role of diagnosis, and its looping effect in the human subject, as described by the philosopher Ian Hacking (1998, 1999), shows how diagnosis and symptoms not only mirror cultural moments in times, but are part of the constitution of the very self who walks into the consulting room. We make sense of ourselves through our belongings, our identifications with a culture or group and its ideas of personhood and self. Foucault (1978) showed us how our internal worlds are themselves caught in power discourses around sexuality and self, and we now have cultural ideas of the self that create depressed, anxious and ADHD young adults arriving at our consulting rooms. Describing their affliction and understanding themselves through unruly brains and serotonin levels, these discourses compete with those of subconscious mysteries and Freudian slips, perhaps even overdetermined by whatever star sign or animal year in which they have been born.

Our idioms of self are intimately related to what anthropology and cross-cultural psychiatry has called our idioms of distress (Nichter, 2010). We can no more interpret these discourses as derivatives of infantile conflicts, primitive anxieties or effective defense mechanisms than we can claim authority over the stories people tell us. Anthropology, psychoanalysis, psychology and even the toa ching all become ways in which people both make sense of their world and constitute their experience. Ethnographies of mental illness finds the prevalence of something we currently all witness in our clinics – where self-diagnosis prevails but within a cultural system where the conceptualization of self has extended to encompass an idea of ourselves as neurochemical functions, coining what sociologist Nikolas Rose (2003) calls "the neurochemical self." Those new subjects who can be medicated and regulated at will to achieve a desired normative functioning (Martin, 2010) all while we psychoanalysts valiantly ask them to consider their internal worlds. Small wonder that in the era of the brain and biology, fantasies of self-transformation remain rooted in the body, from plastic surgery, to tattoos, to medication rather than in the mind.

This most recent wave of anthropological research and ethnographies highlights how expressions of suffering manifest and take shape through idioms – be they centered in the brain, somatic experience, guilt or the collective appearance of new hauntings and idioms of possession (Capley, 2008). If trauma in our western medicalized idioms reverberate through PTSD, trauma in the Other is often experienced as an ontological insecurity brought on through unruly spirit possession (Igreja, 2003; Kleinman, 1986; Pandolfo, 2008). In this framing, the cure is tied as much to the subject of suffering as it is to a biological entity. For the subject, now constituted within different idioms, symptom and cure are intimately intertwined. Possession is not cured in a consulting room. Even schizophrenia or psychosis is differentially experienced in different cultural contexts, which effect both its onset, prognosis and cure (cf. Jenkins and Barrett, 2005). Different versions of the symbolic enable what Ellen Corin (2007) has called positive withdrawal for those with schizophrenia. The advantage for those in some cultural spaces outside of the west lies in the availability of symbols and context that can bind and help the subject understand the Other of psychosis that resides within her. Culture in this sense has been understood to provide a way to make sense of inchoate and unformulated experience – "the work of culture," as Obeyesekere (1990, 1985) argued, is now no longer just a layer above the psyche or epiphenomenal to it, but constitutes the symbolic that can contain, express and even rework pathological experience

Interpretation as the Domestication of Culture

The specter of the Other haunts the scene of our contemporary clinic. Recent psychoanalytic debates embrace difference primarily through a lens of contemporary dynamics encompassing race. Race has come to stand in for the Other in ways that fail to address the different genealogies, histories and thinking that underlie conceptualization of race, as opposed to culture. This conflation further risks universalizing the American racial project and social formation along with its psychological dynamics into a universal fault line. This binary offers a way for the analyst (coded as white) to address and sensitize herself to the discomfort, or vertigo, of misrecognition along with the projection and introjection that occur within the symbolic position of power alongside the racial subjectivity she embodies (see, for example, Layton, 2006). But as race comes to occupy this space of radical difference, culture is tamed. Race provokes anxiety, while the otherness of culture in many analytic writings is understood and captured through a sustained inquiry or impasse to be resolved in moments of revelations, learning and mutual understanding. In this, the culturally aware psychoanalyst explores varied and different cultural dynamics and is sensitive to alternative models of kinship and gender dynamics, power dynamics or to different norms and values (Seeley, 2005). While important, the danger here is that the difference of culture is reduced to competence and sensitivity. The difference emerges and then settles if we listen hard enough, remain open and curious enough, and then as good analysts, we can allow for the difference to reawaken us to our own normative models, just as Ruth Benedict did 100 years ago.

But culture is more than a set of practices, norms and social behaviors to be catalogued as more or less like oneself. Culture encompasses those very symbolic systems that constitute our understanding of self and other. Symbolic systems that can present radically different experiences of self, suffering and experience (above). The demand to interpret or translate this difference, the rituals, religions and healing that seem so far from our own has challenged the anthropologist to address the paradox of how to "interpret" events and beliefs outside of her psychological boundaries and systems of knowledge (Crapanzano, 1980). Anthropology has grappled with its desire to interpret and represent radically different symbolic systems with the knowledge that translation is never innocent. An interpretive method places us at the boundary of understanding and colonization – a danger for psychoanalysts as much as anthropologists. What then can we say about a universal subject if our differing symbolic systems are clashing systems of self understanding? When we encounter radical alterity, a difference that is not just of degree but of symbolic systems, how can the psychoanalyst reconcile our symbolic system with alterity? If psychoanalysis claims an interpretive method, collaborative, intersubjective or one-person, we cannot escape the fact that our hermeneutic for healing and understanding is just one of many symbolic systems. We cannot sidestep the appearance of radical alterity and its translation. This is most evident outside of the west and made clear in with the writings of Frantz Fanon who launched the question of the post-colonial subject, not only challenging previous psychoanalytic descriptions of the colonized, but then theorizing the problem of subjectivity within the gaze of the colonial other (Fanon, 1986). Fanon addresses the violence of interpretation – where he not only insisted on the role of the historical and the socioeconomic context but also addressed the etiology of suffering within the violence of the colonial and psychiatric encounter alongside the subject's search for himself.

Psychoanalysis, regardless of orientation, advocates the dialogic exchange as central to its praxis – whether in the service of uncovering deep unconscious motivation, phenomenological experience in or out of awareness, internalized objects, resistance and defense, or mutual (mis)recognition.[4] If the analyst lays claim to a sensitivity to cultural difference, whatever the difference is, her praxis normally prioritizes interpretation. Even if interpretation can never happen outside of the transference, and the mutative interpretation requires meaning and affect to converge, the anticipation (at least when working with neurotics) is that through the naming of the unsaid, something becomes known that was previously unknown. Individual and dyadic disruption are symbolized and precipitate a subsequent transformation of self-experience. The psychoanalyst awaits the emergence of a reflective agent, a speaking subject, whose life story and experience are explored through a psychoanalytic process that both disrupts rigid narratives and engenders self-knowledge and self-awareness.

In this version, when the subject, or analysand, speaks, she takes up a place within a symbolic system. Our selfhood is taken up within a symbolic system (Crapanzano, 1992). But symbolic systems used to describe psychological experience are referentially varied. A variation reflected at the level of native or local psychological models which constitute different models of subjectivity. Cultures and their symbolic systems provide dramas of self and a coming-into-being. The self-constitution of selves whose world is peopled by spirits and ancestors, whose agency may be determined more by nature and seasons than by internal motivations, is a radically different self-constitution in comparison to the person who believes they are the center of their decision-making. To take these differences seriously asks the psychoanalyst to enter into a space of radical difference. It is easy enough to domesticate experience by translating it into the language of an ego syntonic symptom, or bracketing it into a religious experience to be respected but separate from the psychoanalytic process. Both solutions, one to secularize, the other to paternalize, fail to capture the significance of these differences for the subjectivity of an Other. Psychoanalysis always assumes more than what is said. We assume a hidden, or multiple, meaning for the text and symbols that emerge. We listen for a referential system to be discovered. But what if the differences expressed address the very nature of a hermeneutic in ways that are not easily resolved by interpretation? What is to be done when the experience of profound melancholy over a death produces the haunting by an evil spirit, or cries out with the voices of the dead? When psychological life is not vested in a singular inner experience and the boundaries between self and other are porous as spirits enter and leave the soul? Where life history is not about real versus phantasy but an interaction between persons and non-persons where each represent and symbolize different desires? Where biography is retold as a biography of desire and morality rather than a biography of actual events (Crapanzano, 1980)? In such cases, in what register can or should one interpret – does one look for the truth of history, a traumatic event, symbolic expression of new experiences or a translation of the unconscious? Even Freud came to a place where he said the symbolic would never uncover the full meaning (the navel of the dream). Where do we pitch our interpretation? Towards the basket of failed Oedipal desires and phallic mothers, or into the cruel demons who persecute and dominate.[5]

Conclusion: The Symbolic and the Myth of Psychoanalysis

Psychoanalysis, whether located within the scientific discourse or not, assumes its effectiveness through the symbolic. The talking cure is a cure through symbols by another name. The analyst, in the real or transferential relationship, is constituted within a network of symbolic understandings. An analysand encounters herself and the other through language. She mediates her experience through symbols that remain singular to a subject, overdetermined but representative of internal worlds and unconscious surprises. The subject in an encounter with the symbolic finds new ways to understand and experience, to elaborate a world and remake it at the same time. If our interpretative framework and psychoanalytic hermeneutic has an impact, its effectiveness takes place within a symbolic frame. In this act, the symbolic both represents and transforms simultaneously; the cure that demonstrates the power that symbols have over our internal world (Obeyesekere, 1990).

Psychoanalysis explores a singular subject woven into a symbolic world. In contrast, anthropology has a history of meddling in other worlds where the spiritual and medical are not separate domains. Where symbols and rituals manifest conflicts tied as much to the sociocultural domain as within the individual (Turner, 1975). And, as with the patient's dreamworld that churns up primary process and symbolic solutions, ritual practices create symbolic worlds that enable transformations through new symbolic understandings and embodied experience. Ritual practices operate within ceremonial time and enable liminal spaces that enable social and/or personal change. In these ritual moments, symbols and the worlds they populate are invested with an affective valence and embody multiple meanings that render them more powerful.

If psychoanalysis relies on the hermeneutic interpretation of the overdetermined symptom and its symbolic meanings, were it to enter into a dialogue with anthropology, its cure might be seen to hover within the realm of ritual. In 1949, Claude Levi-Strauss, aware of this congruence, wrote the essay *The Effectiveness of Symbols* (1949a), where he documents the song of the Kuna shaman that enables a woman to overcome a difficult labor. The shaman's incantation begins with long repetitive stanzas that retell the story of the shaman's arrival, returning the woman back to the beginning of her difficult labor and then continues with a song that alternates between the struggle of the shaman and his helpers (represented as figurines) and the spirits in the woman's body. The woman's body and the spirits become interchangeable within the text, as the stanzas flip between them. Levi-Strauss argues that the move in the text from myth to body and back is what enables the cure (where the body, the uterus and the vaginal openings are symbolized s hills and pathways in the incantation). The shaman's song lays out a mythic reality which symbolizes and makes sense of the woman's disrupted experience. One order of experience (the mythic) is mapped onto the other (psychophysiological). For Levi-Strauss, the shaman's song creates symbolic equivalency, a referential text of symbols that relate different orders of experiences back onto each other. There is no direct interpretation, but the woman succeeds in integrating inchoate experiences through this movement from myth to body and back: something happens and the mind and body are reorganized. He is not so interested in the something, the how, nor does he assume one order is bedrock (the body) on which the other (language) acts as would the analyst assume with the hysterical or psychosomatic subject. His position is that new associations between different registers allow for the change.

For Levi-Strauss, the cure is psychological but precipitated through the symbolic. Its effectiveness happens through culturally generated symbols which derive their strength through myth. Much of Levi-Strauss' work was devoted to elaborating the underlying structures of myth, which he argued represent the structure of the unconscious. An unconscious which for Levi-Strauss is what enables and structures the symbolic function. It is this symbolic function that inscribes us into the social. It is what distinguishes nature from culture. In the Kuna song, the cure derives from the (re)inscription of the woman into a social myth. *She finds her place in the symbolic.* At the end of the essay, pivoting to psychoanalysis, Levi Strauss then argues for an equivalence – he proposes that the cure through a social myth with the Kuna is exchanged in psychoanalysis for a cure through the individual myth of the analysand. Change happens through the location of a subject within the mythic – one social and the other individual.

The cure voyages through an unconscious, but this unconscious is not repressed content, or id-based derivatives or experience that remains out of awareness. It is a structure that has the capacity to generate and relate unconscious thought. It is the opposite of a Freudian unconscious that seethes with primary process and unbidden ideas, nor is it the Lacanian unconscious which is structured through language. Levi-Straus proposes something different, that the unconscious is the basis of the symbolic. The building block that underlies all social life. Even if one disagrees with his binary structural determinants of myth (and by now many do), Levi-Strauss takes seriously the power of the unconscious in its capacity to cure. And while endowed with this capacity, it needs the social to set it in motion. In another paper, written in the same year, *The Sorcerer and His Magic* (1949b), the comparison between the shaman and the psychoanalyst is further elaborated as he argues that ritual and its symbolic efficacy, i.e., cure, requires a consensual validation within the social world. The cure will not happen if one does not start with a belief in the cure. Magic, like the placebo, cannot work if there is no belief in it to start. Levi-Strauss proposes a shamanistic complex where a triangle of the social, the shaman and the patient are all implicated in the process, to the point where, "XX did not become a great shaman because he cured his patients, he cured his patients because he was a great shaman – thus we reach the collective pole of our system" (Levi-Strauss, 1949b, p. 174).

For the contemporary psychoanalyst, it is hard not to squirm as we are aligned with the shaman and his magic; to imagine we reside in the *Weltanschauung* that Freud was so eager to leave, and which in western culture would exile us from scientific legitimacy, even though these readings of Levi-Strauss argue against the binary of science and belief to begin with. And yet we cannot fail to know that our discovery of our unconscious process does not emerge from science or study, but from our experiential process, our own analysis, where we bump up against it, sideways, through the Other. We end up believing in it, not proving it. It emerges through a movement from skepticism to belief – and one might argue it emerges through a ritual, where the analyst maintains her belief even when the analysand chafes. Levi-Strauss makes then what might be considered an ethical move – he puts psychoanalysis in the same order as the shaman (Freud of course turning in his grave) and he exposes our own myth, our own symbolic order which keeps medicine and the shaman separate. The later belonging to the order of belief, the former to science. And we know where Freud and his followers feel more at home, less othered. But in this move, Levi-Strauss not only demonstrates the role of the symbolic, he provokes an anxiety about where the psychoanalyst belongs within it, leading many to run for the hills of scientific legitimacy and escape from the valley of belief. While science may indeed have much to teach the analyst, and contribute to her practice, the fear of our own other, of being associated alongside the shaman, evokes the anxiety that the constitution of the psychoanalyst and the register she occupies may indeed owe more to ritual and magic than scientific legitimacy.

While psychoanalysis developed in once eminent institutes, throughout its development, it has generally closed its doors and guarded its boundaries, suggesting an underlying vulnerability. In spite of various attempts, anthropology has only ever been taken up in an ad hoc way by psychoanalysis and certainly never as an intellectual discourse with which to be seriously engaged in spite of a shared inquiry into human variation and experience, whether in the psyche or culture. Levi-Strauss outlines one reason for the unease that may sabotage these attempted dialogues and rendered them invisible – started and then forgotten or repressed. For beyond any institutional arrangements that separated the protagonists, there may be a suspicion, an unformulated anxiety, of what might happen next. A dialogue where anthropology becomes the Other to Psychoanalysis. Where it opens a crack in the wall and puts the narrative at risk. It points to the magic underneath the science, and with this leaves psychoanalysis perched even more precariously within the symbolic system instead of granting it the authority some crave and the legitimacy others seek through the discourse of science, especially in the North American milieu. The divergence that was the beginning of this encounter between the fields suggest an anxiety; the fear is of a dialogue that could initiate a potential dissolution, an opening up of boundaries and a reconstitution of self. And so in its place we are left with the fragments of half-started dialogues that began with Freud and continue with Sapir and Benedict and others after, pieces of a conversations that remain enigmatic, which never quite enter the mainstream. A continual repression of false starts, of conversations that happened before, screen memories of previous beginnings that then disappear maybe precisely so as to leave psychoanalysis feeling safe, if alone, once again.

Notes

1. One of Hall's most notable contribution was his published theory of adolescence in 1904 (Hall, 1904) where he extrapolated a universal theory of psychological conflict and functioning based on the forces of puberty that left a child subject to its competing needs and meant adolescence ushered in a period of "Storm and Stress" (German: Sturm und Drung).
2. For Freud, the subject emerges in the Oedipal phase, along with law (the incest taboo) and therefore culture. The first anthropologist to take this up (and the originator of the anthropological method of participant observation), Bronislav Malinowski (1884–1942), in dialogue with Freud went to the Triobrand Islands to search for the law among the "savage." (Malinowski, 2008) Malinowski not only argued for a complicated law and morality but argued that there was a modified Oedipal structure given matrilineal kinship models, which give authority to the mother's brother (Stocking, 1986b). Such debates were quelled by Jones, and more or less summarily dismissed by the Freudians. But this argument has continued to generate discussions among anthropologists who contemplated how to understand alternative forms of social organizations and governing systems outside of the west (cf. Paul, 1989).
3. Sapir, also a poet, would rework this same problem through poetry, where the singularity of the poet works within the form of the poem. A model that gives vision to his idea of culture and the limits and possibilities it engenders. (Benedict and Sapir, both poets, were to grow in their disagreements over culture, but remained connected through a vibrant correspondence over their poems).
4. Although the non-verbal is increasingly important from some schools, and it is theorized to transcend some social or symbolic mode of representation in most cases, the practice remains that this will be put into language, unless it is assumed to be some form of early mother-infant regulation in the dyad as proposed by some of the Boston Change Group or Jessica Benjamin.
5. One of the most comprehensive projects to address this question was in the Fann Clinic in Dakar Senegal. Run by Henri Collomb, the Ortigues, a psychologist and philosopher worked with patients there and thought about the problem of working psychoanalytically in the post-colonial context. There they address the question of translation and find ways to connect idioms of suffering along with psychoanalytic concepts, such as

the Oedipal structure, as well as considering the different relationship to the body and time that originates from different childhood care and modes of separation (Bullard, 2005, Collingnon, 2018).

References

Benedict, R. (1934). *Patterns of Culture*. Boston, New York: Houghton Mifflin Company.

Benedict, R. (1938). Continuities and Discontinuities in Cultural Conditioning. *Psychiatry: Journal of the Biology and the Pathology of Interpersonal Relations*, 2, 161–167.

Bonovitz, C. (2005). Locating Culture in the Psychic Field: Transference and Countertransference as Cultural Products. *Contemporary Psychoanalysis*, 41, 55–76.

Briggs, J. (1970). *Never in Anger: Portrait of an Eskimo Family*. Cambridge, MA: Harvard University Press.

Bullard, A. (2005). Oedipe Africain: A Retrospective. *Transcultural Psychiatry*, 42, 171–203.

Capley, J. (2008). Haunting Ghosts. Madness, Gender and Ensekerite in Haiti. In M. Delvecchio Good et al. (Eds.) *Postcolonial Disorders, Reflections on Subjectivity in the Contemporary World* (pp. 132–156). Oakland CA: University California Press.

Collingnon, R. (2018). Henri Collomb and the Emergence of a Psychiatry Open to Otherness through Interdisciplinary Dialogue in Post-Independence Dakar. *History of Psychiatry*, 9(3), 350–362.

Corin, E. (2007). The "Other" of Culture in Psychosis: The Ex-Centricity of the Subject. In J. Biehl et al. (Eds.) *Subjectivity: Ethnographic Investigations* (pp. 273–314). Oakland, CA: University of California Press.

Crapanzano, V. (1992). *Hermes' Dilemma and Hamlet's Desire: On the Epistemology of Interpretation*. Cambridge, MA: Harvard University Press.

Crapanzano, V. (1980). *Tuhami, portrait of a Moroccan*. Chicago: University of Chicago Press.

Dimen, M. (Ed.) (2011). *With Culture in Mind*. New York, NY: Routledge.

Foucault, M. (1978). *The History of Sexuality*. New York, NY: Pantheon Books.

Fanon, F. (1986 [1952]). *Black Skin White Masks*. London, UK: Pluto Press.

Fisek, G.O. (2010). Relationality, Intersubjectivity and Culture: Experiences in a Therapeutic Discourse of Virtual Kinship. *Studies in Gender and Sexuality*, 11(2), 47–59.

Frie, R. (2014). What is Cultural Psychoanalysis? Psychoanalytic Anthropology and the Interpersonal Tradition. *Contemporary Psychoanalysis*, 50(3), 371–394.

Freud, S. (1914). *On the History of the Psychoanalytic Movement*. Transl. James Strachey. Standard Edition, Vol. XIV. London: Hogarth, pp. 3–66.

Fromm, E. (1944). Individual and Social Origins of Neurosis. *American Sociological Review*, 9(4), 380–384.

Gaskins, S. (2006). Cultural Perspectives on Infant-Caregiving Interactions. In N. Enfield and S. Levenson (Eds.) *The Roots of Human Sociality: Culture, Cognition and Interaction* (pp. 279–298). Oxford, UK: Berg.

Gottlieb, A. (2004). *The Afterlife is Where We Come From: The Culture of Infancy in West Africa*. Chicago, IL: University of Chicago Press.

Hall, S. (1904). *Adolescence: Its Psychology and its Relations to Physiology, Anthropology, Sociology, Sex, Crime, Religion and Education*. New York, NY: D Appleton and Company.

Horney, K. (1937). *The Neurotic Personality of Our Time*. New York, NY: WW Norton and Co.

Jenkins, J. and Barrett, R. (2005). *Schizophrenia, Culture and Subjectivity: The Edge of Experience*. Cambridge, MA: Cambridge University Press.

Konner, M. (2016). Hunter Gatherer Infancy in the Context of Human Evolution. In C. Meehan and A. Crittenden (Eds.) *Childhood: Origins, Evolution and Implications* (pp. 123–154). Albuquerque, NM: University of New Mexico Press.

Groark, K. (2019). Freud among the Boasians: Psychoanalytic Influence and Ambivalence in American Anthropology. *Current Anthropology*, 60(4), 559–588.

Hacking, I. (1998). *Rewriting the Soul: Multiple Personality and the Science of Memory*. Princeton, NJ: Princeton University Press.

Hacking, I. (1999). *The Social Construction of What*. Cambridge, MA: Harvard University Press.

Hegarty, P. (2005). Harry Stack Sullivan and His Chums: Archive Fever in American Psychiatry? *History of the Human Sciences*, 18(3), 35–53.

Igreja, V. (2003). "Why are There So Many Drums Playing until Dawn?" Exploring the Role of *Gamba* Spirits and Healers in the Post-War Recovery Period in Gorongosa, Central Mozambique. *Transcultural Psychiatry*, 40(4), 459–487.

Irvine, J. (2002). Editor's Introduction. In J. Irvine (Ed.) *Edward Sapir: The Psychology of Culture. A Course of Lectures* Second Edition (pp. 1–22). New York, Berlin: Mouton de Gruyter.

Kenny, R. (2015). Freud, Jung and Boas: The Psychoanalytic Engagement with Anthropology Revisited. *Notes Rec R Soc London*, 69(2), 173–90.

King, C. (2019). *Gods of the Upper Air: How a Circle of Renegade Anthropologists Reinvented Race, Sex, and Gender in the Twentieth Century.* New York, NY: Doubleday.

Kleinman, A. (1986). Social Origins of Distress and Disease: Depression, Neurasthenia, and Pain in Modern China. *Current Anthropology*, 27(5), 499–509.

Lancy, D. (2008). *The Anthropology of Childhood: Cherubs, Chattels and Changelings.* Cambridge, UK: Cambridge University Press.

Layton, L. (2006). Racial Identities, Racial Enactments and Normative Unconscious Processes. *Psychoanalytic Quarterly*, 75(1), 237–269.

LeVine, R. (2014). Between Geertz and Kohut: Chicago in the 1960's. *Clio's Psyche*, 20(4), 443–447.

LeVine, R. (2002). Culture and Personality Studies, 1918-1960: Myth and History. *Journal of Personality*, 69(6), 803–818.

Levi Strauss, C. (1977 [1949a]). The Effectiveness of Symbols. In C. Levi-Strauss *Structural Anthropology* (pp. 186–205). New York: Basic Books.

Levi Strauss, C. (1977 [1949b]) The Sorcerer and His Magic. In C. Levi-Strauss *Structural Anthropology* (pp. 167–195). New York: Basic Books.

LeVine, R. and Norman, K. (2008). Attachment in Anthropological Perspectives. In R. Levine and R. New (Eds.) *Anthropology and Child Development: A Cross Cultural Reader* (pp. 127–142). Malden, MA: Blackwell Publishing.

Mageo, J. (2013). Toward a Cultural Psychodynamics of Attachment: Samoa and US Comparisons. In N. Quinn and J. Mageo (Eds.) *Attachment Reconsidered: Cultural Perspectives on a Western Theory* (pp. 191–214). Palgrave McMillan.

Mead, M. (2008). The Ethnography of Childhood. In R. Levine and R. New (Eds.) *Anthropology and Child Development* (pp. 22–27). Malden, MA: Blackwell Publishing.

Malinowski, B. (2008). Childhood in the Triobrand Islands, Melanesia. In R. Levine and R. New (Eds.) *Anthropology and Child Development: A Cross Cultural Reader.* Malden, MA: Blackwell Publishing.

Molino, A. (2004). *Culture, Subject, Psyche: Dialogues in Psychoanalysis and Anthropology.* Middletown CT: Wesleyan University Press.

Moore, H. (2007). *The Subject of Anthropology.* Cambridge, UK: Polity Press.

Martin, E. (2010). Self Making and the Brain. *Subjectivity*, 3(4), 366–381.

Nichter, M. (2010). Idioms of Distress Revisited. *Culture, Medicine, and Psychiatry: An International Journal of Cross-Cultural Health Research*, 34(2), 401–416.

Obeyesekere, G. (1990). *The Work of Culture: Symbolic Transformation in Psychoanalysis and Anthropology*. Chicago, IL: University of Chicago Press.

Obeyesekere, G. (1985). Depression, Buddhism and the Work of Culture in Sri Lanka. In A. Kleinman and B. Good (Eds.) *Culture and Depression: Studies in the Anthropology and Cross-Cultural Psychiatry of Affect and Disorder* (pp. 134–152). Oakland, CA: University of California Press.

Pandolfo, S. (2008). The Knot of the Soul. Postcolonial Conundrums, Madness, and the Imagination. In In M. Delvecchio Good et al. (Eds.) *Postcolonial Disorders, Reflections on Subjectivity in the Contemporary World* (pp. 328–358). Oakland CA: University California Press.

Paul, R. (1989). Psychoanalytic Anthropology. *Annual Review of Anthropology*, 18, 177–202.

Peters, M. (2010). Culture as Self Object and Its Impact on the Self. *Psychoanalytic Inquiry*, 30, 357–367.

Quinn, N. (2013). Adult Attachment Cross-Culturally: A Reanalysis of the Ifaluk Emotion Fago. In N. Quinn and J. Mageo (Eds.) *Attachment Reconsidered: Cultural Perspectives on a Western Theory* (pp. 15–39). NY, New York: Palgrave McMillan.

Reiss, B. (2005). The Subject of History/The Object of Transference. *Studies in Gender and Sexuality*, 6(3), 217–240.

Rose, N. (2003). Neurochemical Selves. *Society*, November/December, 46–59.

Sapir, E. (2002a). The Patterning of Culture. In J. Irvine (Ed.) *Edward Sapir: The Psychology of Culture. A Course of Lectures* (pp. 103–123). New York, Berlin: Mouton de Gruyter.

Sapir, E. (2002b). Psychological Aspects of Culture. In J. Irvine (Ed.) *Edward Sapir: The Psychology of Culture. A Course of Lectures* (pp. 175–190). New York, Berlin: Mouton de Gruyter.

Sapir, E. (1938). Why Cultural Anthropology Needs the Psychiatrist. *Psychiatry: Journal of the Biology and the Pathology of Interpersonal Relations*, 1, 7–12.

Sapir, E. (1937). The Contribution of Psychiatry to an Understanding of Behavior in Society. *American Journal of Sociology*, 42, 862–870.

Sapir, E (1934) The Emergence of the Concept of Personality in a Study of Cultures. *Journal of Social Psychology*, 5, 408–415.

Seeley, K. (2005). The Listening Cure: Listening for Culture in Intercultural Psychological Treatments. *The Psychoanalytic Review*, 92(3), 431–452.

Roth Pierpoint, C. (2004). The Measure of America. Annals of Culture. *The New Yorker*, March 1, p. 48.

Stocking, G. (1986a). *Malinowski, Rivers, Benedict and Others: Essays on Culture and Personality*. Madison, WI: University of Wisconsin Press.

Stocking, G. (1986b). Anthropology and the Science of the Irrational: Malinowski's Encounter with Freudian Psychoanalysis. In G. Stocking (Ed.) *Malinowski, Rivers, Benedict and Others: Essays on Culture and Personality* (pp. 13–49). Madison, WI: University of Wisconsin Press.

Turner, V. (1975). Symbolic Studies. *Annual Review of Anthropology*, 4, 145–161.

Chapter 3

More Simply Human Than Otherwise

Interpersonal Psychoanalysis and the Field of the "Negro Problem"

Michelle Stephens

Early in 1939, Harry Stack Sullivan found himself in Greenville, Mississippi, commissioned to perform a psychoanalytically informed study of American race relations. The request came in 1938 from his colleague, Charles S. Johnson (1893–1956), then a leading black sociologist at Fisk University who would go on to become the President of Fisk (Rose, 2005, p. 338). While at Fisk, Johnson was joined by another prominent African American scholar, E. Franklin Frazier (1894–1962), and they would both publish key texts in black sociology at the beginning of the 1940s. Johnson published *Growing Up in the Black Belt: Negro Youth in the Rural South* in 1941 while he was leading the Department of Social Sciences at Fisk, and Frazier published *Negro Youth at the Crossways: Their Personality Development in the Middle States* in 1940, while leading the Department of Sociology at Howard. Both works included writing by Harry Stack Sullivan. Sullivan's "Memorandum on a Psychiatric Reconnaissance," a reflection on his time in Mississippi, appeared as an appendix in Johnson's work, and his discussion of the case study of a young black man, given the name Warren Wall, accompanied Frazier's chapter on the subject.[1] By 1940, the year Sullivan's First William Alanson White Memorial Lectures were published in *Psychiatry*, he was also in the midst of significant scholarly and personal interaction with colleagues and interview subjects, both black and white, on the question of race in the United States (see Ursano, 2012).

Just before that, in February of 1938, Sullivan had consolidated his sense of the necessity of interdisciplinary study for the mental health field by founding the journal *Psychiatry: Journal of the Biology and Pathology of Interpersonal Relations*. The journal explicitly stated its commitment

DOI: 10.4324/9781003270355-4

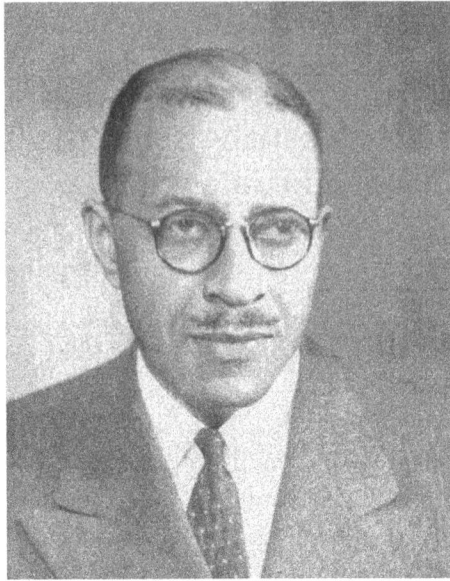

Figure 4 Charles S. Johnson, 1947, © Fisk University, John Hope and Aurelia
        E. Franklin Library, Special Collections, Fisk Photograph Collection.

to publishing the work of "all serious students of human living in any of its aspects" (William Alanson White Psychiatric Foundation, 1938, p. ii). As the editors of this collection point out, the four issues of the journal's first volume were led by a cross-disciplinary mix of scholars, including a psychiatrist, a political scientist, an ethnologist, and a psychoanalyst. Their interdisciplinary mixture both derived from and supported a larger scholarly investment in a vision of the human rooted in the cultural and the social rather than in the natural and the biological.

As Sullivan sat in the pantry of Walker Percy's uncle's home in Greenville, Mississippi, he was also sitting right at the heart of the interpersonal psychic and social field of American racial relations. As the poet pithily described the scene:

> Dr. Sullivan's methodology: Early each afternoon he made himself a pitcher of vodka martinis—no one had ever heard of such a drink in Mississippi in the 1930s—and set up shop in the pantry, listened and talked to any and all comers. I never did find out what this brilliant and sardonic upstate New Yorker made of race relations in Uncle Will's pantry.
>
> (Percy, 1991, pp. 65–66)

For all of its seemingly casual charm, everything about Sullivan's unusual "consulting room" for these interviews was both psychologically and methodologically meaningful. "The white folks in the front," friends and neighbors of the Percys who were interviewed, arrived through the dining room. Black subjects, "the cook and her friends and friends of the cook's friends in the back," arrived through the kitchen (Percy, 1991, pp. 65–66). Sullivan, the only other person 'working' in the home alongside the cook, placed himself in the pantry, a space connected with but also subordinate to both the kitchen and the dining room, a space of both residence and work, domesticity and professionalism. There he drank his vodka martinis and, under the cover of sociability, attempted to learn what he could about the impact of race on "human living" (William Alanson White Psychiatric Foundation, 1938, p. ii).

This unorthodox setting was essentially a "field" in two senses of the word, one specific to the disciplinary context of Sullivan's psychoanalytic research in the late 1930s, and the other more relevant for the twenty-first century. For the 1930s, describing his time spent in Will Percy's Greenville home as time in the field refers to the new priority that was being placed on fieldwork in the South among a group of researchers in the social and mental sciences, the "human sciences" as Rose terms the disciplines collectively, who were Sullivan's contemporaries and compatriots (Rose, 2005, p. 338). This interracial group of scholars included the sociologists Johnson and Frazier, but also, white sociologist John Dollard and anthropologist Hortense Powdermaker. Both published their own psychosocial studies of race relations during this period, *Caste and Class in a Southern Town* (1937) and *After Freedom* (1939). And all were invested in participant-observation as a foundational method and practice for gathering data, which meant they actually travelled to the south to try to talk to black and white subjects as the source of their scholarship. The need for fieldwork was demanded by their theory—that if interactions between people and events give meaning to those people and events, to understand the impact of race on human living, they would need to observe racialized and interracial interactions within their cultural settings by being *a part* of them, by being *participants*. In the late 1930s of Sullivan's visit to the South, fieldwork was a necessary feature of a developing psychosocial methodology linking the mental and social sciences.

The second relevant notion of the field is more contemporary and involves the broader ways in which Sullivan brought "field theory" to psychoanalysis. In his discussion and overview of a number of psychoanalytic field theories, Donnel Stern describes how Sullivan drew from the embryological and biological sciences as much as the social sciences in crafting his notion of a field of interactive events. The field was less an explicit focus in Sullivan's work and more a product of his foregrounding of interaction and relatedness. As Stern describes more fully:

> The concept of the field…is simply that the analytic situation is defined in terms of its relatedness. Analyst and patient are continuously and inevitably, and consciously and unconsciously, in interaction with one another. This interaction has to do with what they experience in one another's presence, and how they behave. The field also determines what each participant can experience in the presence of the other, especially the affective aspects of experience. The field is, on one hand, the sum total of all those influences, conscious and unconscious, that each of the analytic participants exerts on the other. On the other hand, the field is the outcome of all those influences, the relatedness and experience that are created between the two people as a result of the way they deal with one another.
>
> (Stern, 2015, p. 35)

In Stern's and most strictly psychoanalytic understandings, the "field" is limited to and defined by the interaction between two persons. For social theorists, and for a psychoanalytic contemporary of Sullivan's such as Erich Fromm (1994), the sociocultural and the political always precedes the interpersonal and is the ground out of which interpersonal interaction emerges and takes place. Since Sullivan never made explicit his thinking about the structure of the social field and its bearing on psychoanalysis, it is not clear that he would have gone as far as Fromm.

In the writings Sullivan produced during 1938–1941, however, specifically those discussing antiblack racism and antisemitism that are the focus here, what is clear is that Sullivan was interested in the process by which racial attitudes become personal and *interpersonal*, that is, deeply inflecting, and inflected by, human social relations. In the early 1930s, as Rose also explains using language from the period: "'[t]he true locus of culture is in the interactions of specific individuals' and 'in the world of meanings which each one of these individuals may unconsciously abstract for himself from his participation in these interactions,'" and culture and society were "the sum of interpretive acts" (Rose, 2005, p. 323).[2] This chapter argues that precisely what Sullivan contributed to the study of the broader sociocultural "field" of "the Negro Problem" in early twentieth century US history was an approach to *how*—and what, where and why—the individual "may unconsciously abstract for himself from his participation in these interactions," that is, make racial meaning in a space, or field characterized by the social and the personal, and enacted in the interpersonal. "Fieldwork," then, is used intentionally to place both of these senses of the word side by side, describing Sullivan's research methodology on the one hand, but also, using his writing to think about the psychoanalytic dimensions of the broader field of American race relations as it interacted with, and continues to interact with, the more strictly two-person field of interpersonal psychoanalysis. Between Fromm's notion of social character and the psychoanalytic focus on the individual psyche, stood Sullivan's and his peers' focus on personality, and their efforts to study the interpersonal and sociohistorical fields in which personalities are formed.

This chapter reflects on Sullivan's fieldwork in the 1930s southern and mid-states, performed at the same time and in dialogue with his November 1938 editorial on anti-Semitism in *Psychiatry*, and the relevance of all three writings for thinking psychoanalysis and race together in our contemporary moment. Sullivan's editorial, memorandum, and discussion of Warren Wall's case study together provide material for a reflection on what Sullivanian psychoanalysis had the potential to offer the study of, and clinical practice within, the field of American race relations. That racial field included a scholarly sub-field, the disciplinary and interdisciplinary interactions and relations that constituted the late 1930s and early 1940s emergent community of black and white researchers, psychiatrists, and writers thinking about the interracial problem of 'the Negro' and about human encounters across racial lines.

The Field of Personality

Both the social and mental health sciences in the 1930s were undergoing a profound paradigm shift in how researchers understood the foundations of human nature. Harry Stack Sullivan was very much a part of this shift. As Robert J. Ursano describes: "Sullivan saw humans as primarily social beings and was interested in how the individual's social and cultural environment affected inner life" (Ursano, 2012, p. 1). Sullivan's time in Greenville was explicitly to study "the effects of race on personality development" (Ursano, 2012, p. 1). Personality, the keyword in these discussions, was conceived of as "the subjective outcome of social experience and a force in society in turn," and was the relevant phenomenon that "situated the individual in culture" (Rose, 2005, p. 323). This seemingly straightforward definition had significant repercussions for thinking about race in the late 1930s and early 1940s.

In Sullivan's 1938 editorial on anti-Semitism in *Psychiatry*, it is his notion of what it means to *personalize* history that stands out, helpful even for thinking about contemporary race relations (see Sullivan, 1938). Recounting the centuries-old history of anti-Jewish sentiment in Christianity, Sullivan emphasized the psychodynamic context in which symbolic language, discourse, ideology—social discourses— interact with individual subjects' specific histories. Even social forces occur in dyadic contexts, as he asserts in his very opening line when he states: "Hatred is an attitude of a person involved in interpersonal relations" (Sullivan, 1938, p. 593). His second line extends this point one step further—"Unpersonalized objects and abstractions are not hated. Collectivities of people are hated only in so far as they are embodied in concrete personalizations or personifications." A subject positions a collective in their mind as a hated object through acts of "personalization," through specific memories, events, attachments, salient for and in their own personal history. Even as they originate from the social, these "personalizations" are deeply unconscious and specific, "uncommunicable, quite beyond consensual validation" (Sullivan, 1938, p. 593). As Sullivan theorized further: "In the study of personality...the more troublesome of one's me-you patterns.... Unfolds itself as a dynamism that was evolved in an inevitable fashion in the individual's concrete life experience. The origin of each personalization is seen to have been *historically necessary*" in the life of the individual (Sullivan, 1938, p. 595). Racism, racialism, in the individual has a developmental history: "From its origin in concrete experience and a real interpersonal situation, each personalization has itself had a developmental history" (Sullivan, 1938, p. 595). Such a history is analyzable, if the analyst cares to attend to these particular personalizations.

While he gestures in his editorial to thinking comparatively about anti-Catholic and "antinegro prejudices" or "anti-negroism" alongside anti-Semitism, Sullivan hit a wall when he faced 'the Negro problem' head on in the deep south (Sullivan, 1938, p. 595). Struck by the levels of violence and the conditions of both psychic and physical fear African Americans lived within, he tried to contextualize his lack of success in making real contact with black southerners: "I did not succeed in establishing contact with any of those who were described by my informants as 'just average [Negroes].' I learned in the first few days that I could not bridge the cultural gap with most of the plantation workers. The Negro seems to have a notably great capacity for sensing by intuition interpersonal reality" (Sullivan, 1963, p. 179). As a participant-observer engaged in fieldwork in this very specific, racialized, historical field,[3] Sullivan walked away from Greenville "intellectually shaken" by what he experienced there (Rose, 2005, p. 322). His letters from Mississippi to Charles S. Johnson reveal his despair at the "holocaust" in the "Deep South"—"'the abysmal lack of opportunity' for black youth and their inability to trust" (Rose, 2005, p. 322). In his striking use of the term 'holocaust,' years before it would take on the specific historical reference to the genocidal policies and actions of the Nazis against Jewish people during World War II, Sullivan was pointing to the excessive levels of trauma and primal anxiety operative between the black and white races in particular in 1930s America, and profoundly formative in shaping American personalities for generations before and to come.[4] His own participation in this realization, however, was not a scientifically or psychoanalytically detached one, but rather, *personally* destabilizing and traumatizing, as he also revealed in his private correspondence: "I am a damned fool to expect to understand anything much about human personality" (Rose, 2005, p. 322). While in this same period he also collaborated with E. Franklin Frazier in studying black male youth from a different region of the country than the South, he went no further in bringing his brush with the American dilemma of race more centrally into his theory of an interdisciplinary, psychoanalytic, psychosocial mode of psychiatric inquiry.

While hitting that wall, however, or maybe because of it, Sullivan's impressions as laid out in the two pieces he wrote about his experience in the field, as he was launching *Psychiatry*, offer a set of crucial formulations very much in dialogue with his discussion of anti-Semitic personalizations. In his memorandum included in Johnson's study, despite a first paragraph suggesting that "nothing of optimistic expectation as to results was developed from his trip down south," he proceeds in his very next paragraph to make a key distinction between two forms of racism:

> Throughout my work with marginal individuals, I have heard a variety of all-inclusive generalizations about the Negro group. In work with persons representative of more privileged American society, I have observed the coexistence of these generalized beliefs with contradictory individualized thinking and behavior towards members of this group. The 'logic-tight compartment' principle is conspicuous here. It appears that the generalized (often derogatory) belief is an essential part on one's emotional make-up, whereas the more valid individual formulations are much less emotionally significant.
>
> (Sullivan, 1963, p. 175)

In this seemingly simple, but actually quite dense, passage, first Sullivan notes that anti-black racist thoughts among Americans tend to take two forms, "all-inclusive generalizations" based on little to no experience with black people, and "contradictory individualized thinking and behavior towards members of this group." One can imagine that, among the white southerners he sat, drank, and chatted with, pleasant and affectionate interactions with black members of their staff sat side by side with virulently racist attitudes about African Americans more generally. In referencing the "'logic-tight compartment' principle," Sullivan borrows a term from evolutionary biology also used by the English psychiatrist W. H. Rivers in 1920 to describe dissociation:

> All of us in some degree, and many persons in a high degree, keep their beliefs and thoughts in separate compartments which have been called 'logic-tight compartments.' In these cases, each of two sets of beliefs or thoughts is accessible to the other, but no effort is ever naturally made to bring them into relation with one another. The special feature of these cases is a failure of fusion or integration which brings them definitely into relation with dissociation.
>
> (Rivers, 2012, p. 83)

Sullivan's third observation is that what helps to maintain this form of dissociation, this inability to stand in the spaces between dissociated states and to observe and to link them to each other, is *not* the emotional salience of the specific experiences one has with members of a group one feels prejudice towards. These would be the type of real-life experiences one might have in interracial settings, in workshops on cross-cultural communication, etc. Unfortunately, the former remain disconnected from the emotional depth of the "generalized (often derogatory) belief[s that are] an essential part on one's emotional make-up" (Sullivan, 1963, p. 175). Derogatory generalizations learned in the past, in other words, continue to hold more psycho-emotional resonance than relations or attachments that might contradict those generalizations in the present. The "emotional make-up" Sullivan references here links to what he describes in his editorial on anti-Semitism as a personalization or personalized object, tied to important events and meaningful attachments in the subject's past. These racist, "logic-tight compartments" operate much like the notion of a bastion in contemporary psychoanalytic field theory.[5] Created, *personalized*, in one's familial and social context, in the interactions, acts of interpretation, symbolization, meaning-making, and unconscious fantasies, that occupy a bi-personal field, bastions can only be pried apart in the context of an analysis that unravels the strands of interpersonal anxiety, obligation and trauma that led to the creation of a past bastion, and its analytic re-enactment.

Sullivan's second important observation in "Memorandum of a Psychiatric Reconnaissance" is one that may seem more obvious now, until one defamiliarizes the present by reminding ourselves of the state of scientific research on the black subject relevant in 1938 when Sullivan was writing. As Rose reminds us, by the 1930s, understanding of the black mind was still governed by a somatic scientism, that is, "a blend of biological and evolutionary assumptions" that "arranged groups defined by somatic traits on a progressive scale" (Rose, 2005, p. 323). The most benevolent racist attitude such an approach generated was paternalism, as reflected in Howard Odum's 1910 work, *Social and Mental Traits of the Negro*, in which the black subject's ability to 'know himself,' to 'comprehend the essential weaknesses of the race,' would "induce whites to behave toward compliant blacks with 'tolerance, broadmindedness and patience.'" Not surprisingly, "Caucasian brains," in contrast, "showed 'will power, self-control, self-government,' while Negroes [] were 'affectionate, immensely emotional, then sensual and under stimulation passionate'" (cited in Rose, 2005, p. 329). "Black character, to whites, was synonymous with weakness" as evident in "a stream of publications around 1900 about the race's mental disorders." It was precisely these attitudes that Sullivan and his friends and contemporaries, such as Edward Sapir, a Yale anthropologist who was also one of the founding editors of *Psychiatry*, attempted to shift away from with their broader focus on culture.

It is clear that Sullivan was writing very pointedly against these older notions in "Memorandum of a Psychiatric Reconnaissance." His black subjects shared no obvious traits, no inherent weaknesses, or even anything that was distinctively "black." Rather, what black Americans shared was a trauma, one Sullivan described very intentionally as an *interracial* rather than a racial trauma, that is, a trauma constituted out of and within the interracial interpersonal field, not a trauma somehow inherent to a damaged black psychology. It was the social situation that was traumatic, and the black subject bore the burden of that trauma. As Sullivan summarized his observations: "In a few words, it was easy to discover not one general type but very wide differences of personality among Negro youth in the southern area. It is impossible to find much of anything that is unique or general in American Negro personality, excepting only an almost, if not quite, ubiquitous fear of white people. These interracial attitudes always came to the front" (Sullivan, 1963, p. 175). Shifting to a brief case, Sullivan told the story of an encounter with a young black man that bore out his theory regarding the personalization of generalizations, embedded in deep personal, cultural, psychosocial histories, which sustained themselves with a rigidity and intractability above and against the experience of relational interaction in the present.

Recounting what one might also describe as the transferential dimensions of the interracial field, Sullivan shared: "one of my three best informants in this area shocked himself by realizing belatedly that he was telling me how deeply he hated all whites. Here, too, we seem to have a generalization essential to the self; again, one that is no barrier to quite contradictory specific beliefs and behavior. This particular young man was quick and accurate in perceiving the nuances of our relationship, and, aside for this one instance of painful embarrassment, expressed himself with rather astonishing freedom from restraints"

(Sullivan, 1963, p. 175). Sullivan was describing the deeply dissociative structure of racial generalizations, as personalizations created out of past trauma as opposed to traumatic racial relations in the present. The young man was experiencing what Rivers called in 1920 a "co-consciousness" as much as something unconscious, that is, less something sitting underneath than something sitting alongside, and what W. E. B. Du Bois called a condition of "double consciousness" specific to the African American situation (Rivers, 2012, p. 75; Du Bois, 1994, p. 2).

Anne Rose has offered a very useful account of the broader scholarly context Sullivan was operating within. The very inter-disciplinarity that produced the journal *Psychiatry*, for a brief moment in the late 1930s and early 1940s, also came close to allowing a research method profoundly informed by interpersonal psychoanalytic modes of inquiry to tell a different kind of cultural story about race in America. This was one in which blackness and whiteness were not seen as discrete categories, racial cultures with separate traits that require intercultural communication, but rather, as elements in a shared, interpersonal, social dynamic with a history, and with personal implications for the various American personalities operating within this field. In her clarifying and deeply archival account, Rose describes a series of figures who essentially, as they attempted to process what they encountered down south, were forced to adapt older social and mental science models in order to deliver a psychosocial analysis that had features we can also recognize in Sullivan's work.

However, according to Rose, many of these figures got caught between the Charybdis of academic marginalization and the Scylla of race reform politics. Either their research on race relations specifically was not objective or scientific enough for many of the foundations sponsoring the work, or, as Du Bois, one of the most prominent black intellectual elders of the time, criticized the work of John Dollard, the scholarship was not political enough, was seen as not able or even intended to make a direct intervention in the traumatic social and psychic situation researchers were observing, participating in, and describing. Many of the interracial research partnerships that came out of this 1930s moment ended with the black scholars feeling dissatisfied with their white colleagues' over-reliance on analysis and caution regarding using scholarship to effect social change (Rose, 2005, p. 344). These criticisms obscured what was truly radical about what they were doing, engaging in a form of praxis that tested the limits of a related set of disciplines' understandings of the human subject, and in the very action as much as the recording of their fieldwork, suggesting another way of being human.

The Field of Black Rage

In his "Memorandum," Sullivan mentions another informant with whom "an abortive experiment in more intensive psychiatric study was undertaken," a young man he also suggested exhibited "schizophrenic forms of mental disorder" (Sullivan, 1963, p. 176). As he described their interaction in Mississippi:

> In one, whom unforeseen accident had but recently thrown out of a vassalage relationship with a white plantation supervisor, [he] rapidly focused on the re-creation of such a situation with me. Beginning as a fleeting fantasy that he expressed among several 'thoughts' about the immediate future, I was able to observe its progression to a resolve to break with everything familiar to him and trust his fate to me—all this with no expression of emotion.
> (Sullivan, 1963, p. 176)

The phenomenon Sullivan experienced would be used as the basis of a whole theory of colonial dependent personality a little over ten years later by the French psychoanalyst Octave Mannoni (Mannoni, 1990).[6] Where Sullivan and Mannoni differed, for good or ill, is in the fact that Sullivan did not take the role the young man wished to cast him in, nor did he define their interpersonal dynamic as characteristic of the group of black southerners as a whole. He relates the young man's move to New York, where at first he "showed good capacity for controlling the anxieties that the actual transition included" (Sullivan, 1963, p. 176). However, as his prospects decline and emotional stability deteriorates, it is clear the subject's difficulties have little to do with the quality of his mind, and more to do with the reality of his social condition. Sullivan describes in a footnote,

> The boy of the experiment had an effective formal education amounting to a good second grade, an intelligence that would have carried him through at least junior high school. His career

had encouraged him to but little curiosity about events external to his narrow personal horizon. He had, however, rather firm ideals as to working for a living which, too, suffered in the debacle of the northern translation, in no small part, doubtless, because of my inability to assume a useful role in the transitional phase. I was away most of the time on the study in a border area.

(Sullivan, 1963, p. 176)

The study Sullivan references was his second engagement with the interracial situation of young black Americans and race relations during this same period. He agreed to consult on E. Franklin Frazier's *Negro Youth at the Crossways*, a study of black adolescent personality development, which Sullivan describes in his "Memorandum" as, "An intensive psychiatric study of a few American Negroes of northern urban habitat" (Sullivan, 1963, p. 175). This study produced a third writing on race in this period, his discussion of the case of "Warren Wall," a young man not from the south but from the border states closer to the north who was part of the group participating in Frazier's study (see Sullivan, 1940).

Warren Wall, as E. Franklin Frazier described him, was "a tall, lithe, well-built, dark-brown boy of sixteen with an intelligent face and pleasing personality, [who] appears to be a serious youth. He seldom smiles when talking, uses no gestures, and generally gives the impression that he is getting information rather than giving it" (Frazier, 1940, p. 205). What made him stand out for Sullivan was "the success of his discriminating me as a person from 'the white man' as a generalized object of hostility" (Sullivan, 1940, p. 229). Warren Wall relied less on projection and more on his experience in his generalizations regarding Sullivan, the white psychiatrist. Whereas in the earlier study in the south, the affect Sullivan was most struck by among African Americans was fear, regional comparison allowed him to identify rage as the more relevant affect for black Americans living in the north. The shapeshifting nature of racism in the United States had a concomitant, variegated impact on black personalities.

Throughout his discussion of Warren Wall's case, Sullivan demonstrates an informed understanding of the impact of class and sexual dynamics on Warren's sense of freedom. He observes, for example, both "that the 'promiscuity' in sexual relations and the 'superficiality'

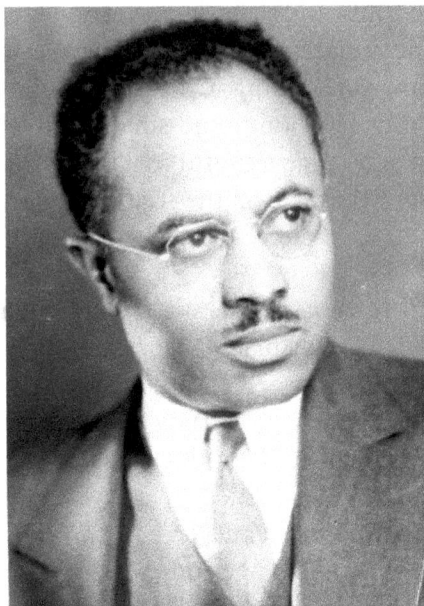

Figure 5 E. Franklin Frazier, 1938, © Moorland-Spingarn Research Center, Howard University Library.

in friendship relations arise from a complex of traits that we would refer to a frustration in elaborating the *good-mother preconcept"* (Sullivan, 1940, p. 231). Too fleeting for a psychoanalysis proper, Sullivan's comments do reflect some of the starting elements of a possible psychoanalytic cultural criticism, that is, the interdisciplinary analysis of race's intersection with culture using the theoretical tools of psychoanalysis.[7] What stays relevant psychoanalytically is his characterization of all of Warren Wall's relevant behaviors, attitudes, complexes, as due to interracial factors having to do with the "haphazard" nature of discrimination in the border states, as compared to the systematic discrimination of the south.

In Warren Wall, Sullivan saw less a black subject who was "subconsciously made to be chronically afraid" than one who had been "ignored and treated with indifference or frank contempt" (Sullivan, 1940, p. 231). Warren's regional corner of the American interracial social field operated differently than the "distance-fixing etiquette and caste-distinguishing system of taboos of the southern regions" (Sullivan, 1940, p. 231). Precisely what that difference produced was a different impact on personality, on the emotional channels and defenses through which black subjects managed the affects produced from, originating in, their socio-racial context. And whereas the systematic discrimination of the south produced in black subjects, such as the young man who briefly found refuge in New York, a soul-crushing fear that sought escape in fantasy or in reality, the more northern patient felt rage: "The border Negro struggles with rage where the southern Negro suffers from fear. The unconstructive wish-fulfilling fantasies that are evoked by these states are respectively malevolent and escapist" (Sullivan, 1940, p. 233).

For Sullivan, the "tragedy of the Negro in America" was an interracial phenomenon; it had an interpersonal, relational source that was also a "vicious circle" (Sullivan, 1940, p. 234). Once again and even more firmly in this piece, he countered the general racist consensus of his field:

> In serious discussion of this problem with highly intelligent and ordinarily resourceful confreres, I have been told in essence that there doubtless are unusual Negroes, but that it takes a psychiatrist interested in the problem to find them. I have heard much about 'typical Negro characteristics' and, unhappily, when my role has been commonplace...I have had experiences that could be readily rationalized in accord with these 'typical characteristics.'
> (Sullivan, 1940, p. 233)

Here Sullivan then performed a bit of important self-analysis, asserting: "However, when the role is shifted and the techniques of intensive study of interpersonal relations have been substituted for those of a detached and generally preoccupied professional man, the presumptively 'typically Negro' performances have been resolved into particular instances of the 'typically human.'" Sullivan the "preoccupied professional" white man was as susceptible to his own personalized generalizations about the black "citizens of our commonwealth" (Sullivan, 1940, p. 234). Sullivan the interpersonal, psychoanalytic psychiatrist called on his colleagues to cultivate within themselves "a humanistic rather than a paternalistic, an exploiting, or an indifferent attitude" and charged the mental field itself to take responsibility for its own neurotic projections: "As a psychiatrist, I have to speak particularly against using them as scapegoats for our unacceptable impulses; that fact that they are dark-skinned and poorly adapted to our historic puritanism is really too naïve a basis for projecting most of our privately condemned faults upon them. They deserve to be observed as they are, and the blot of an American interracial problem may thus gradually be dissipated" (Sullivan, 1940, pp. 233–234).

In the early twentieth-century period in which Sullivan was writing, there were no outpatient services for black subjects. "Any care outside custodial institutions for the black mentally ill, or, for that matter, for whites, was a rarity in the South" where as many as two-thirds of black families lived (Rose, 2005, p. 329). So one has to wonder, what did the Warren Walls and southern black boys Sullivan met do with all of the fear and rage that was and continues to be a part of their American existence? For as both Anne Rose and Beverly Stoute retrace, over much of the twentieth century and even now into the twenty-first, both psychoanalysis and psychiatry have failed the black subject (Rose, 2005, p. 329; Stoute, 2017).[8] Indebted to a certain notion of the psychoanalytic subject, the self, it has at best incorporated a notion of the black as Other without questioning the very terms on which the notion of the human is constructed. What happens, then, to those Frank Wilderson calls "too black for care," lost in "so much anxiety" and "bereft of a critical race vocabulary" (Wilderson, 2020, p. 17).

Sullivan's observations about both the black mind and the interracial field, many of which flew in the face of much of his psychiatric contemporaries' thinking, would all appear in fleshed out form in the writing of black authors before, during, and after, the years 1938–1940. The story did not end with Sullivan, in other words, but to the detriment of psychoanalysis and psychiatry, the rich, interdisciplinary space of cross-over and interaction between scholarly fields did close up, and with negative consequences for psychoanalytic thinking. As Stoute laments: "racism, subtle and overt, has impeded the development of psychoanalysis as a theory and as a field of practice forestalling our further understanding of race, racialization and racism" (Stoute, 2017, pp. 28–29). Thus as late as 1999, over 60 years after Sullivan's founding of *Psychiatry*, there were still only twenty-six African American members of the American Psychoanalytic Association (Stoute, 2017, p. 18). To gain a sense of the complexity of the black internal, and external, experience then, one would have to turn to black literary writing and culture by some of the most power-ful African Americans writers, such as Toni Morrison.

Even in Sullivan's time, as early as the nineteenth century slave nar-ratives, black subjects have been working through the traumatic real-ities of America's interpersonal interracial field in their imaginative works, putting their "wish-fulfilling fantasies" on paper (Sullivan, 1940, p. 233). The southern young black man Sullivan encountered and describes in "Memorandum on a Psychiatric Reconnaissance," whose dream to move north failed, shared a story and an experience with the title character of the 1953 National Book Award-winning novel *Invisible Man*, and with the author of that novel himself, Ralph Ellison. Serendipitously, when Ellison first moved north in 1936, he found work, temporarily, as Sullivan's receptionist, and when Sullivan wrote recommendation letters for the young Ellison, little did he know that years later, that very trope of the white patron of the black male migrating north would make its way into Ellison's defining American novel. In *Invisible Man,* the supposed positive letter of reference from a white patron turns out to be a hoodwink, one that keeps the protagonist running fruitlessly in place till he col-lapses in a despairing retreat from the social world. Ellison's invisi-ble man was an alter ego of Sullivan's southern patient, who found himself back home when no one, including Sullivan, could help him fulfill his fantasy of a successful transition to the north. And both the southern boy in New York and Warren Wall, the mid-state black subjected to indifference, could find an alter ego in the main pro-tagonist of the even more contemporaneous 1940 novel, Richard Wright's *Native Son*, the story of a young black man who falls victim to his own dissociated, murderous black rage, the novel itself playing out a malevolent black psychotic fantasy.

The black subjects in Frazier's, Johnson's, and Sullivan's studies could also have found parts of themselves, parts of a shared expe-rience, in Richard Wright's memoir, *Black Boy*, published in 1945, which told the story of his own youth in the south, in Mississippi, Arkansas, and Tennessee and his move north to Chicago. If Sullivan, briefly, served as Ellison's white mentor, Wright was Ellison's black mentor, introducing him to the literary worlds of Chicago and New York. In this same period and on into the 1950s, both Wright and Ellison would become intensely involved in the psychiatric world by collaborating with the German and Marxist psychoanalytic psychiatrist, Fredric Wertham, in opening the Lafargue Mental Hygiene Clinic in Harlem in 1946.[9] Wright would describe the situation of blacks in New York and the mental health clinical field very bluntly in his 1946 essay "Psychiatry Comes to Harlem," where he linked the country's lack of a real commitment to actualizing African Americans' entitlement to mental health care in the north to a similar lack of commitment to actualizing their vote in the south:

> [T]hat Harlem's 400,000 black people produced 53% of all the juvenile delinquents of Manhattan, which has a white population of 1,600,000; that, while in theory Negroes have access to psychiatric aid (just as the Negroes of Mississippi, in theory, have access to the vote!), such aid really does not exist[,] owing to the subtle but effective racial discrimination that obtains against Negroes in almost all New York City hospitals and clinics; that it is all but impossible for Negro interns to gain admission to hospitals to receive their psychiatric training.
>
> (Wright, 1946, p. 50)

These were some of the dynamics linking the political, the psychiatric, and the psychic in the shared interracial field of 'the Negro problem' in the mid-twentieth century United States. The field also revealed its global and postcolonial extension when, in 1953, a young Caribbean psychiatrist, Frantz Fanon, wrote to Richard Wright about his novel *Native Son* and memoir *Black Boy*, on the heels of publishing his own psychoanalytic work, *Black Skin, White Masks*. While in residency in psychiatry at Saint-Alban-sur-Limagnole in France, Fanon trained under another Marxist psychiatrist, Françoise de Tosquelles, who in the European context pioneered the idea of socio-therapy or socio-analysis with an emphasis on the role of culture in psychopathology. Fanon would bring this sensibility, as both a clinical and institutional methodology, to his own tenure as *chef de service* at the Blida-Joinville Psychiatric Hospital in Algeria.[10] In this series of encounters, black writers and psychoanalytic thinkers of the mid-twentieth century were drawn to psychoanalysis and psychiatry because of their own experiences in a global, interpersonal, social field created by colonialism and racial slavery, that stretched across the black Atlantic world between Europe, Africa, and the Americas. It was these men and their female peers who carried on, in their prose and creative writings, the work of understanding race and race relations as an interpersonal mental field embedded in the sociocultural, and personalized through the psychic, an approach whose relevance Sullivan first got a sense of from his own interactions with black Americans. Beverly Stoute asks poignantly, "Did the unexamined racism of how people of color were viewed and othered, even by analysts, silently stifle our development as a field?" (Stoute, 2017, p. 28). The brevity of this moment of interdisciplinary and interracial interaction in these fortuitous two years between 1938 and 1940, between such scholars and 'fieldworkers' as Sullivan, Johnson, Frazier, Powdermaker, and Dollard, the fleeting nature of their intersection with such black imaginative thinkers and writers as Ellison and Wright, represents one such lost opportunity for the field. Instead, the playing out of the psychic and unconscious dimensions of the interpersonal field of American race relations, the theorizing and conceptualizing, observation and reflection, on its manifestations from a near-experience, here and now position, became an imaginative subject for African American literature and a critical topic of analysis in the broader field of African Diasporic cultural studies.

As Sullivan, Frazier, and Johnson were writing about black boys in the south and mid-states, writers such as Wright and Ellison were describing their own, personal, versions of that experience in the journey from South to North, and reframing their histories in fiction. What fiction allowed was not simply insight into black interiority, although it did and does provide that. Black fiction, poetry and prose writing—the black literary imagination—was also a site for the black subject to pursue, speculate, inquire into, the difficulty white subjects seemed to have in just seeing blacks as fellow humans, and relatedly, to express, voice, symbolize, and thereby manage their personal sense of indignation at the social, interpersonal, and existential conditions of their existence as a result of that social fact. Throughout his writing career, Wright engaged imaginatively in his own kind of psychosocial inquiry into both the black and white mind based on the lived experience of his interracial interactions. The methodology was humanistic, using a fundamental belief in the power of human imagination to question both the natural and the human orders as constructed. And the process of discovery, the psychic excavation of this American interracial field, often produced rage.

Many years later, in 1968, African American psychiatrists William Grier and Price Cobbs named at least one of the primary affects Sullivan discerned from his interviews of 1938, black rage. Another five decades later, in the wake of a racial epidemic that included police killings of black men, disproportional incarceration of black people, and the equally disproportional impact of the Covid 19 global pandemic on African American and Latinx American front-line workers, Beverly Stoute has challenged the psychoanalytic and psychiatric fields, once again, to understand black rage as a structuring element of an interracial, interpersonal, American field. As she asserts:

> *'Rage'* [is] 'a deeply rooted emotional reaction to a perceived injustice that differs from anger...' and one that 'is directly and poignantly linked to experiences with degradation, marginalization...devaluation [and oppression].' *Black rage* builds up as an accumulated adaptive reaction to experiences of racism and discrimination over generations.... *Black rage* is contextualized, therefore, in African American culture and defined as operative in the sustained response of oppressed people who endure repeated acts of injustice without opportunity for redress.... *Black rage*, if mobilized in a functional way, can have a specific cultural, transmutative, adaptive potential.
>
> (Stoute, in press)

Key to Stoute's formulation is the pairing of black rage with moral injury, the latter as theorized by Jonathan Shay. For Shay, the "betrayal of what is right either by a person in legitimate authority or by one's self in a high stakes situation.... Impairs the capacity for trust and elevates despair, suicidality, and interpersonal violence" (cited in Stoute, in press). This betrayal, which impairs one's sense of one's own dignity, produces an 'indignant rage' against "a violation of what's right" (cited in Stoute, in press). Stoute's crucial insight is that, rather than a rage with unfettered bounds, black rage as moral injury has been precisely an adaptive mechanism that bridges between the psychic and political, turning moral outrage into a useful, life-affirming, *personalization* of the racist psychodynamics of the American interpersonal interracial field, into a re-invocation and reminder of one's own humanity in the face of social death.

The mechanisms, the forms of this mode of psychic adaptation, the moral injury and black rage as precisely the *personalization* of the American interracial experience, are all examples of the psychic phenomena that Beverly Stoute argues the psychoanalytic field would benefit from analyzing. If psychoanalysts wish to make sustained contact with the interpersonal interracial field within which we practice, such an analysis is crucial. For what is black rage but a response to the specific experience of being ousted outside of the boundaries of the human, which no academic discourse, no philosophy, no human science of the twentieth and twenty-first century has been able fully to name and acknowledge, much less historicize and explain—except for black studies.

The Field of the Human

The quirkiness of Percy's "quaint tale" of Sullivan's studies of interracial relations in the South does not reflect the more serious impact of this visit on Sullivan, as detailed by Anne C. Rose (2005, p. 321). For Rose, "The truth was more ragged," and if anything: "Personality as an idea, embraced as the perfect synthesizing tool, worked a bit too well when it brought the depth of racial problems into focus" (Rose, 2005, p. 321). Percy, brushing off the visit as not allowing for enough time (three weeks in total) for Sullivan to produce any comprehensive analysis, was unable to see that the informal, odd setting was precisely what would have given Sullivan a strong, personal, analytic, impression of the field in which he was a participant-observer. As Sullivan himself described, he was there as the analyst, not simply the professional or the researcher. And as such, setting a frame around his sitting area in the pantry he would have known that its unconscious borders were porous, that he was integrated in, rather than detached from, the field of his interactions. Despite Walker Percy's memory, Sullivan was not a house guest of the Percy's. His own domicile during his stay was at a room at the Hotel Greenville. For all of Sullivan's studied casualness, his sessions in the pantry were a space for work and consultation. Instead, it was from his own private space at the Hotel Greenville that Sullivan wrote Johnson of the profound despair he experienced as a result of these sessions and encounters.

What he could not know, but we analysts of the twenty-first century have access to both in the canon of African American literature and in the sophisticated theorizing of black analysts, such as Stoute and Grier and Cobbs before her, is that black despair and the performance of infra-humanity does not just end there. Rather, it leads to a rage that needs to be managed, sublimated. Black literature and creative acts of imagination have provided a powerful, consistent, vitalizing way of managing that rage, with a sense of moral injury that is its own validation and the sign of a psychic life and "aliveness" that still manages to persist, despite the realities and constraints of black social death.[11] For Wilderson, "'Mad at the world' is Black folks at their best," empowered and emboldened with "the freedom to say out loud what we would otherwise whisper or deny: that no Blacks are in the world, but, by the same token, there is no world without Blacks" (Wilderson, 2020, pp. 39–40). That aliveness was a resource that crystallized into the civil rights movement, and that aliveness is very much with us again in the era of Black Lives Matter.

For a range of contemporary black studies scholars and writers, it is now clear that a central structuring element of the field of black studies scholarship and writing in the Americas, from its origin in the early slave narrative to the present moment, has been the pursuit, and expression, of alternative understandings of the human.[12] Using a more humanistic methodology, these black humanists have tried to follow the path of the human sciences, even as psychoanalysis and psychiatry have abandoned exploring the psychic impact, good and bad, of both an existential and an ontological splitting off of black people from our common sense understandings of the human—what Sullivan described as the "community of assumptions," what we all can assume we "know []...to expect" about what it means to be human. This leaves the black subject, "the Negro, well trained in the almost infra-human role," as Sullivan saw in 1938 (Sullivan, 1940, p. 233), with a profound experience of oneself as "the foil of Humanity," as Wilderson is still describing almost a century later (Wilderson, 2020, p. 13).

It was precisely in an effort to theorize the black experience of infra-humanity that, in 1952, the black psychiatrist Frantz Fanon would assert: "Freud insisted that the individual factor be taken into account through psychoanalysis. He substituted for a phylogenetic theory the ontogenetic perspective. It will be seen that the black man's alienation is not an individual question. Beside phylogeny and ontogeny stands sociogeny.... Let us say that this is a question of a sociodiagnostic" (Fanon, 1986, p. 13) For Fanon, his sense that "Man is what brings society into being" was necessary for black psychic survival (Fanon, 1986, p. 13). For the Caribbean philosopher Sylvia Wynter, understanding our notions of the human as derived, in any given era, from a sociogenetic principle means that "our present mode of sociogeny, the way we at present normatively know Self, Other, and social World" is no more or less true than "the mode of sociogeny of medieval latin-Christian Europe" (Wynter, 2003, p. 269). Just as humans have created genres of literature, so too have we created genres of the human that are realized in the intersubjective fields that comprise hierarchical social structures. Wynter's genres of the human are like Sullivan's generalizations, but now raised to the level of a higher ontological principle.

What does it mean to locate the origin of the human in the social, the sociogenetic? For many black thinkers, it means everything we think we know about what it means to be human is a construction, embedded in a history of colonial modernity built on the exclusion of black being. This profound exclusion of black being, founded in slavery, is the field of the human we all inhabit—scratch the surface of how you think about the human and the exclusion of black subjects will lie somewhere, unconsciously, there, disavowed. This is the radical 'pessimism of the intellect' Afropessimist Frank Wilderson III challenges both psychoanalytic and social theory to wrestle with. For Wilderson, black rage is itself the celebration of black life: "Black people were the living, breathing contradistinction to life itself, And when we were too old...or were too young [to know better], we refused the ruse...and let our rage speak the truth: Human life is dependent on Black death for its existence and for its coherence" (pp. 41–42). When he asserts that slavery was a relational dynamic—think Sullivan's interracial field—and that the very paradigm of the human has to be rethought, he describes us as living our humanity as a bastion of modernity, in a shared unconscious fantasy that occupies almost any bi-personal field, requiring a psychoanalysis that can engage in the dismantling of that paradigm through the praxis of calling the episteme into question as it manifests itself in the personal relationship and interactions between analyst and analysand.

This essay has been an opportunity to think about the Sullivanian notion of the field as exemplified in his field work of 1938–1940, its relevance for discussions of race at mid-century through the notion of personality, its place in dialogue with the work of contemporaneous black thinkers and writers, and its implications for thinking about the human. As Rose says succinctly, "Sullivan came south to learn about human beings" (Rose, 2005, p. 322). Sullivan was part of the field that laid the "intellectual and psychological groundwork of civil rights," but he was also part of the moment in which "controversy at home propelled retreat from the field" (Rose, 2005, p. 325). When the mental and social sciences retreated from the symbolic and cultural field and back toward the 'hard' sciences, they lost the humanistic understanding that all knowledge created by and within the human context is a sociogenetic act. This was one of the true insights of inter-personal psychoanalysis' cultural, social, and intellectual milieu, as "part of a broad, cross-disciplinary movement to recast society as a uniquely human product" (Rose, 2005, p. 323). This is also what black studies has been articulating across the twentieth century landscape of theories of the human, challenging our most fundamental episte-mological and ontological frameworks. In their praxis, Sullivan and his colleagues endeavored to realize Sullivan's vision that we are all 'more human than otherwise,' but not by determining that we are all the same. Rather, in his own fieldwork, he came to learn that there were more versions of what it means to be simply human than what was captured in his personal and psychoanalytic philosophy.

Notes

1. Sullivan's "Memorandum on a Psychiatric Reconnaissance" was first printed as an Appendix in Johnson's *Growing Up in the Black Belt* (1941). The version quoted here was reprinted as chapter 19 in *Mental Health and Segregation: A Selection of Papers and Some Book Chapters*, edited by Martin M. Grossack (1963), 175–179. Also see, "Discussion of the Case of Warren Wall," in Frazier, *Negro Youth at the Crossways* (1940), 228–234.
2. Rose is quoting from Yale anthropologist Edward Sapir's "Cultural Anthropology and Psychiatry" (1932), reprinted in David G. Mandelbaum (1949), ed., *Selected Writings of Edward Sapir in Language, Culture and Personality* (p. 15).

3. In his editorial on anti-Semitism, Sullivan (1938) describes the psychiatrist's role in these terms: "psychiatry is the study of the interpersonal relations in which one integrates oneself as a participant observer" (p. 597).

4. Others, including the editors of this collection, have pointed to Sullivan's distinctive usage of the term 'holocaust' in this specific context. For historian Anne Rose and psychoanalyst Ira Moses, in their direct interpretation of Sullivan's letter to Johnson in which he uses the word, Moses believes "Sullivan was saying it would take a 'holocaust' to clear up the race problem. What is incredible about this word use, according to Rose (personal communication), is that the word 'holocaust' was not used to describe the extermination project toward the Jews until a decade or so later. That makes his word usage that much more powerful and original." Personal communication with Ira Moses, February 2nd, 2021. Clearly, as Sullivan himself suggests by attempting to think about anti-Catholic prejudice, antiblack racism, and antisemitism, side by side, it is the *virulence* of racially violent attitudes and interactions, with deeply traumatic impacts on personality, that associatively connected these forms of racial and ethnic hatred in Sullivan's mind as devastating social phenomena requiring catastrophic, holocaust-like, solutions.

5. For more on "bastions" or "bulwarks," see Baranger and Baranger (2009) and Stern's (2015, pp. 76–79) discussion of "Enactments and bastions." For more on "logic-tight compartments," see contemporary writings by Michael Shermer, columnist for *Scientific American* between 2001 and 2019, https://michaelshermer.com/sciam-columns/logic-tight-compartments/, accessed January 20th, 2021.

6. For more, see Octave Mannoni's *Prospero & Caliban: The Psychology of Colonization* (1950; 1990); for a strong critique of Mannoni's analysis of a dependent personality among the inhabitants of Madagascar, see Frantz Fanon, *Black Skin, White Masks* (1986).

7. See my discussion of the work of both the African Americanist theorist Hortense Spillers on a psychoanalytic cultural criticism, and of the German psychoanalyst Alfred Lorenzer on a cultural psychoanalytics, in "Alfred Lorenzer, Black Lives Matter, and a Cultural Psychoanalytics for Our Times," forthcoming.

8. See Beverly J. Stoute's comprehensive tracing of psychoanalysis' study of 'the Negro,' often very much *not* within the framework of a transferential field of race relations, in "Race and Racism in Psychoanalytic Thought: The Ghosts in Our Nursery," *The American Psychoanalyst*, Vol. 51, No. 1, Winter/Spring 2017.

9. For the authors' own accounts of their involvement with the Lafargue Clinic, see Richard Wright's "Psychiatry Comes to Harlem" (*Free World*, September 1946, pp. 49–51) and Ralph Ellison's "Harlem is Nowhere," written in 1948 but not published until 1964 in his essay collection *Shadow*

and Act. For more contemporary accounts, see Badia Sahar Ahad's *Freud Upside Down: African American Literature and Psychoanalytic Culture* (2010) and Chapter 4, "'The Possibility of Love': Black Psychoanalysis from Harlem to Algeria" in Daniel José Gaztambide's *A People's History of Psychoanalysis: From Freud to Liberation Psychology* (2019).

10. For more on Fanonto:te the editacharya\\Desktop\\Cenveo\\D, see Gaztambide (2019), who also describes his correspondence with Richard Wright, and David Marriott (2018), *Whither Fanon?: Studies in the Blackness of Being.*

11. For more on black aliveness and the power of the black imagination as precisely one of these forms of psychic adaptation, see Quashie (2021). For more on black social death, see Patterson (1982) and JanMohamed (2005).

12. Alexander Weheliye makes this point explicitly when he describes the centrality of "the intellectual project of black studies vis-à-vis racialization and the category of the human in western modernity" (p. 3). As he continues: "Some scholars associated with black and critical ethnic studies have begun to undertake the project of thinking humanity from perspectives beyond the liberal humanist subject, Man.... The greatest contribution to critical thinking of black studies—and critical ethnic studies more generally—is the transformation of the human into a heuristic model and not an ontological fait accompli (p. 8). [*Habeas Viscus: Racializing Assemblages, Biopolitics, and Black Feminist Theories of the Human* (2014)].

References

Ahad, B. S. (2010). *Freud Upside Down: African American Literature and Psychoanalytic Culture.* Champaign, IL: University of Illinois Press.

Baranger, M. and Baranger, W. (2009). *The Work of Confluence: Listening and Interpreting* in the Psychoanalytic Field. Ed. *L. G. Fiorini.* London: Karnac Books.

Dollard, J. (1937). *Caste and Class in a Southern Town.* New Haven: Pub. for the Institute of Human Relations by Yale University Press.

Du Bois, W. E. B. (1903/1994). *The Souls of Black Folk.* New York: Dover Publications, Inc.

Ellison, R. (1952). *Invisible Man.* New York, NY: Random House.

Ellison, R. (1964). *Shadow and Act.* New York, NY: Random House.

Fanon, F. (1967/1986). *Black Skin, White Masks.* Trans. Charles L. Markmann. New York: Grove Press Inc., 1967; London: Pluto Press, 1986.

Frazier, E. F. (1940). *Negro Youth at the Crossways: Their Personality Development in the Middle States.* Washington, D.C.: American Council on Education.

Fromm, E. (1994). "Appendix: Character and the Social Process." In *Escape from freedom*. New York: Henry Holt and Company.

Gaztambide, D. J. (2019). *A People's History of Psychoanalysis: From Freud to Liberation Psychology*. New York, NY: Lexington Books.

Grier, W. and Cobbs, P. (1968). *Black Rage*. New York: Basic Books.

JanMohamed, A. R. (2005). *The Death-Bound-Subject: Richard Wright's Archaeology of Death*. Durham, NC: Duke University Press.

Johnson, C. S. (1941). *Growing Up in the Black Belt: Negro Youth in the Rural South*. Washington, D.C.: American Council on Education.

Lorenzer, A. (1986). "In-Depth Hermeneutical Cultural Analysis." Trans. Katharina Rothe, Daniel Rosengart and Steffen Krüger. *Originally published in Tiefenhermeneutische Kulturanalyse*, Ed. Alfred Lorenzer. Kultur-Analysen. Frankfurt/Main: Fischer. 7–112.

Mandelbaum, D. G. (1949). (Ed.) *Selected Writings of Edward Sapir in Language, Culture and Personality*. Berkeley, CA: University of California Press.

Mannoni, O. (1990). *Prospero & Caliban: The Psychology of Colonization*. Trans. Pamela Powesland. Paris: Editions de Seuil, 1950; Ann Arbor, MI: The University of Michigan Press, 1990.

Marriott, D. (2018). *Whither Fanon?: Studies in the Blackness of Being*. Stanford, CA: Stanford University Press.

Odum, H. (1910). *Social and Mental Traits of the Negro: Research into the Conditions of the Negro Race in Southern Towns*. New York, NY: Columbia University Press.

Patterson, O. (1982). *Slavery and Social Death*. Cambridge, MA: Harvard University Press.

Percy, W. (1991). *Signposts in a Strange Land: Essays*. Ed. Patrick Samway. New York, NY: Farrar, Straus.

Powdermaker, H. (1939). *After Freedom: A Cultural Study in the Deep South*. New York, NY: Viking Press.

Quashie, K. (2021). *Black Aliveness, Or a Poetics of Being*. Durham, NC: Duke University Press.

Rivers, W. H. R. (2012). *Instinct and the Unconscious, A Contribution to a Biological Theory of the Psycho-Neuroses*. London: Forgotten Books.

Rose, A. C. (2005). "Putting the South on the Psychological Map: The Impact of Region and Race on the Human Sciences during the 1930s." *The Journal of Southern History*, 71, 321–356.

Shermer, M. https://michaelshermer.com/sciam-columns/logic-tight-compartments/.

Shay, J. (1994). *Achilles in Vietnam: Combat Trauma and the Undoing of Character*. New York, NY: Maxwell MacMillian International.

Shay, J. (2014). "Moral Injury." *Psychoanalytic Psychology*, 31, 182–191.

Spillers, H. (1996). "'All the Things You Could Be by Now, If Sigmund Freud's Wife Was Your Mother': Psychoanalysis and Race." *boundary* 23, 75–141.

Stephens, M. (forthcoming). "Alfred Lorenzer, Black Lives Matter, and a Cultural Psychoanalytics for Our Times." In "In-Depth Hermeneutical Cultural Analysis." Trans. Katharina Rothe, Daniel Rosengart and Steffen Krüger. Originally published in *Tiefenhermeneutische Kulturanalyse*, Ed. Alfred Lorenzer. Kultur-Analysen. Frankfurt/Main: Fischer. 1986.

Stern, D. (2015). *Relational Freedom: Emergent Properties of the Interpersonal Field*. New York, NY: Routledge.

Stoute, B. J. (in press). "Formulating *Black Rage* as a Mobilizing Force during the 2020 Pandemic." *Journal of the American Psychoanalytic Association*.

Stoute, B. J. (2017). "Race and Racism in Psychoanalytic Thought: The Ghosts in Our Nursery." *The American Psychoanalyst*, 51, 10–29.

Sullivan, H. S. (1938). "Antisemitism." Editorial Notes. *Psychiatry: Journal of the Biology and the Pathology of Interpersonal Relations*, 1, 593–598.

Sullivan, H. S. (1940). "Discussion of the Case of Warren Wall." In E. Franklin Frazier. *Negro Youth at the Crossways: Their Personality Development in the Middle States*. Washington, D.C.: American Council on Education, 228–234.

Sullivan, H. S. (1963). "Memorandum on a Psychiatric Reconnaissance." In *Mental Health and Segregation: A Selection of Papers and Some Book Chapters*. Ed. Martin M. Grossack. New York: Springer Pub. Co, 175–179.

Ursano, R. J. (2012). "'More Simply Human Than Otherwise': Harry S. Sullivan's 'Conceptions of Modern Psychiatry', The First William Alanson White Memorial Lectures (Published 1940). Editor's Note." *Psychiatry: Interpersonal and Biological Processes*, 75, 1–2.

Weheliye, A. (2014). *Habeas Viscus: Racializing Assemblages, Biopolitics, and Black Feminist Theories of the Human*. Durham, NC: Duke University Press.

Wilderson III, F. (2020). *Afropessimism*. New York, NY: Liveright Publishing Corporation, W.W. Norton & Company, Inc.

William Alanson White Psychiatric Foundation (1938). Mission Statement. *Psychiatry: Journal of the Biology and the Pathology of Interpersonal Relations*, 1, ii.

Wright, R. (1940). *Native Son*. NY: Harper & Brothers.

Wright, R. (1945). *Black Boy*. NY: Harper & Brothers.

Wright, R. (September, 1946). "Psychiatry Comes to Harlem." *Free World*, 49–51.

Wynter, S. (2003). "Unsettling the Coloniality of Being/Power/Truth/Freedom: Towards the Human, After Man, Its Overrepresentation—An Argument." *The New Centennial Review*, 3, 257–337.

Chapter 4

The Philosophical Foundations of Interpersonal Psychoanalysis

Albert Dunham Jr. and Racial Politics

Pascal Sauvayre

The inaugural issue of *Psychiatry* is characterized by its wide cross-disciplinary range of articles, from anthropology and political science to business organization and socioeconomics, and of course, psychiatry and psychoanalysis. Amongst this heterogenous group, Harry Stack Sullivan (1938) chooses to highlight only one article in his editorial: "In this issue, the longer study is in the realm of philosophy. Dr. Albert Maillard Dunham Jr. presents a searching analysis of the conceptions of futurity and polarity in events. The use of tensional terms is both frequent and necessary in psychiatric formulation of the dynamic type. This study should contribute greatly to their clarity of reference" (p. 143).

Even against the cross-disciplinary standards of the journal, Dunham's article appears to be an outlier. The "Concept of Tension in Philosophy" is a dense philosophical essay, more than twice as long as any other article in the issue. Dunham's paper would, without doubt, fit naturally in a conventional philosophy journal. In his editorial remarks, Sullivan points out that this is Dunham's doctoral dissertation in philosophy, written under John Dewey, the well-known pragmatist philosopher at the University of Chicago.

Notwithstanding the inter-disciplinary aspirations of *Psychiatry*, how did a lengthy article on philosophy find its way into the inaugural issue? As Sullivan suggests in his editorial, the inclusion of Dunham's article is intended to establish the philosophical foundations for a concept central to all human motivation, experience, and action, to the mind, and hence to his own concept of interpersonal relations, and to his thinking more generally as we will come to see. Indeed, Sullivan later refers to this article in the opening chapters of *The Interpersonal*

DOI: 10.4324/9781003270355-5

Theory of Psychiatry (1953, p. 35, ff. 4) as key to understanding his own concept of tension, and in turn anxiety, which will be explored here as the nodal concept for his entire system of thought and practice. This chapter will suggest that the positioning and prominence given to this article, with its explicit reliance on American philosophers, can be interpreted to be part of Sullivan's own attempt to ground the Interpersonal school on solid 'American' philosophical ground as a counterpoint to the Freudian domination of psychoanalysis.

An even more intriguing feature of this article, one that Sullivan may, or may not, have been cognizant of, is that it was not just part of the 'American' philosophical tradition, but of the 'African American' philosophical tradition. While it is clear that Sullivan knew the author was African American, there is no evidence to suggest that Sullivan was significantly aware of African American philosophy. To what extent is African American philosophy distinct from American philosophy more generally? Which of these traditions did Dunham Jr. best represent, and how is that related to the philosophical foundations of interpersonal psychoanalysis? And finally, is the relationship between philosophy and interpersonal psychoanalysis significantly different from the relationship between philosophy and Freudian psychoanalysis?

This chapter will explore Dunham's paper with an eye to its ramifications for psychoanalysis, and examine how Sullivan took this fundamental concept of 'tension' in a very different direction from Freud's. While the concept of tension eventually translates to libido for Freud, Sullivan makes the link to anxiety as a foundational force in 'human living'. But we are left with an intriguing question. If Sullivan highlighted this paper as part of the foundations of his own thinking in American philosophy, why would he include a relative unknown philosopher for that purpose? This discussion will proceed in stages: it begins with a brief biographical account of Dunham, followed by an examination of the tradition of "African-American philosophy". Then the place of philosophy in psychoanalysis is considered before Dunham's philosophy and its relevance for Sullivan's interpersonal theory of anxiety is examined. It will be argued that Sullivan uses Dunham's paper to lay the foundations of his unique and groundbreaking interpersonalist system of thought. My aims are to help the reader appreciate Dunham's work and to reflect on the reasons why his ideas have been so woefully neglected.

Albert Millard Dunham, Jr.: African American Philosopher

Albert Millard Dunham, Jr. (1903–1949) was in fact a rising star in the field of philosophy.[1] His intellectual pedigree could not be more impressive. He obtained his Ph.D. at the University of Chicago under John Dewey and George Hebert Mead, and he had previously studied under Alfred Whitehead at Harvard, all leading philosophers who fully supported his work. As a true American philosopher, he was on track to becoming a full professor at the University of Chicago and one of its most promising young faculty.

But Dunham ran into a wall, a multifaceted wall. Despite a healthy enrollment for his classes, more than half of the students dropped out

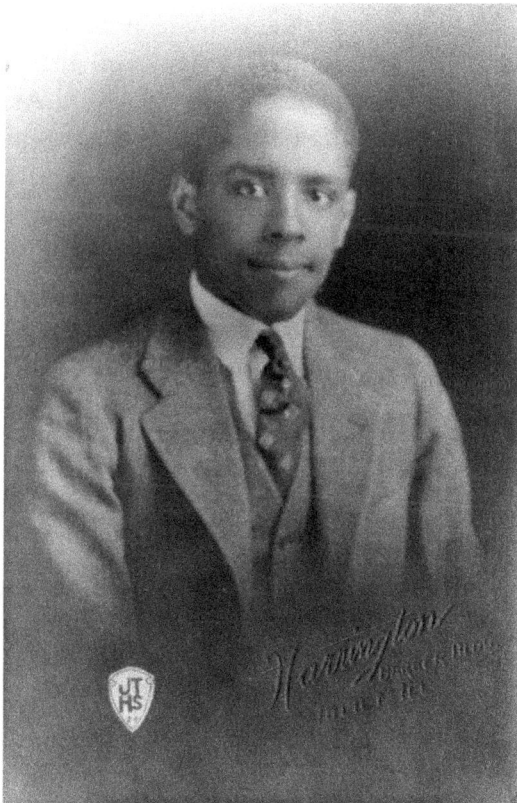

Figure 6 Alfred Dunham Jr. 1926, at age 23, © Missouri Historical Society Photographs and Prints Collection

after the very first class. Unknown to the students when they enrolled, but evident in the first class is, Dunham was Black. At the time there were only three Black scholars with Ph.Ds. serving on the faculties of white universities (McClendon & Ferguson, 2019), and the idea of promoting Dunham along a tenure track was all too quickly abandoned. After leaving Chicago, Dunham would go on to teach at Howard, a historically Black university (HBCU), under the eminent African American philosopher Alain Locke.

Eventually, Dunham died tragically at the very young age of 46 in a psychiatric institution. Those who knew him, including his sister Katherine Dunham (herself a dancer of international renown), thought that his declining mental state was to be blamed on the effects that racism had on his career, which was such a central feature of his identity (McClendon & Ferguson, 2019, p. 39). Indeed, in the words of one of Dunham's contemporaries, William Fontaine wrote in 1944, "The mind of the Negro scholar … is a historical phenomenon, existent in and subject to the influences of its epoch. … As a Negro, the scholar has faced discrimination against his race, and his experiences consciously and unconsciously have engendered psychoses centering around fear, rage, repression, status, and equality. As undergraduate and graduate student, he learns that certain kinds of knowledge lend support to race discrimination" (Fontaine, W., in Harris, 1983, p. 90).

It might be interesting to compare Dunham's trajectory to that of his internationally recognized sister Katherine Dunham (1909–2006), who had an illustrious career as a dancer and choreographer, even earning dozens of honorary degrees. Albert and Katherine were the two children of Fanny (née Taylor) and Albert Dunham. The elder Albert was the descendant of slaves and Fanny of French-Canadian descent. They lived in the Chicago area, and after Fanny's death (Albert Jr. was 9, Katherine was 3), Albert settled in the predominantly white suburb of Joliet, running a dry-cleaning business. Like Albert Jr., Katherine Dunham studied at the University of Chicago, where she eventually submitted her thesis for a Master's Degree in Anthropology, studying with such luminaries as Edward Sapir and Bronislav Malinowski. She showed much promise in academia (Harrison & Harrison, 1999). Katherine Dunham abandoned the world of academia to focus on what turned out to become a highly successful career as a dancer, choreographer, teacher, and social activist.

She was one of Sullivan's more famous patients, and this may have been one of the reasons that Sullivan became interested in Dunham Jr.'s work - this and the fact that she had a romantic relationship with Erich Fromm, who suggested to Sullivan to let her stay in his empty house (Friedman, 2014, p. 93). The success of her career is in sharp contrast to her brother's, "who was considered by many, at that time, to be one of the most promising among African American philosophers to rise in the profession" (McClendon & Ferguson, 2019, p. 38).

As an African American artist, Katherine Dunham had many more opportunities as an artist than her brother did in the context of academia, where "academic racism, the practice associated with the complex of institutions such as colleges and universities, including the posture of the American Philosophical Association (APA), which together function and assert institutional power by erecting standards that, under the guise of professionalization, were and are racist" (McClendon & Ferguson, 2019, p. 38). We can use Freud's perspective on philosophy here. For Freud, philosophy is part of an evolutionary progress that brought human thinking out of religion (and closer to science; see below). If so, then the philosopher descends from the priestly class, and 'he' - of course - therefore carries, like Plato's notion of the philosopher-king, the power that is associated with those who shape, or articulate, our ideology - something we can imagine to be intolerable to most of Dunham Jr.'s University of Chicago students.

In contrast, Katherine Dunham may not have had to face the same kind of racism as an 'entertainer', a domain in which Black performers, if they abided by certain kinds of restrictions that fit the prejudices of white supremacy, were permitted limited 'success'. As Isabel Wilkerson (2020) demonstrates clearly, African Americans could only excel in "the realm carved out for them" by the white caste, and this was as "entertainers and athletes" (p. 137). In the 1930s, "only 5% [of African Americans] were listed as white-collar workers - many of them ministers, teachers, and small business owners who catered to other black people" (p. 135) - one of these being Albert Dunham Jr., one of only *three* black scholars with Ph.Ds. teaching in white universities in 1936 (McClendon & Ferguson, 2019, p. 40).

The entertainer, like the jester, performs for the pleasure of the powerful, and however much a performer can insert subversive content into their performances, they can easily be sidelined into oblivion when the truths they reveal are too uncomfortable for the powerful. And, when the performer steps 'out of line', out of the lines of entertainment and sports they are 'assigned', and into the domain of politics for instance, they are quickly reminded of their 'rightful' place. This phenomenon was recently made evident on a national platform when the NBA star LeBron James commented on the political situation in 2018. Laura Ingraham's comments on Fox News' "The Ingraham Angle" (2/16/18) quickly made national headlines. Adapting her well worn line from her book *Shut Up and Dance* (2006; Regnery, Washington DC), which is intended to keep people she does deem worthy out of the political discourse, she used her racist rhetoric to apply the line to James, telling him to dribble instead. Indeed, this is something that Katherine Dunham could probably attest to when she was arrested by the Chicago police after the 1968 riots that followed the assassination of Martin Luther King Jr. for encouraging local youth to come to her Performing Arts Center to express their feelings and frustrations creatively. This brought national attention and she was quickly released, but it can only have been a clear-cut reminder of the approved 'lines' she could not step beyond.

But there is an even darker side to this that relates to the historical roots of the stereotype of the Black entertainer. As Isabel Wilkerson suggests, the stereotype of the entertaining happy black person finds its roots in the fact that slaves were

> forced to cosign on their own degradation, to sing and dance even as they being separated from spouses or children or parents at auction. 'This was done to make them appear cheerful and happy,' wrote William Wells Brown, a speculator's assistant before the Civil War, whose job it was to get the human merchandise into sellable condition. 'I have often set them to dancing,' he said, 'when their cheeks were wet with tears.'
>
> (Wilkerson, 2020, p. 137)

Wilkerson continues (p. 137), "African-Americans would later convert the performance role that they were forced to occupy". In contrast, by his simple presence in a conventionally white university, Albert Dunham was making the claim to be a 'serious' academic philosopher, on white territory. I would maintain that it was in and of itself a statement of resistance and subversion against white supremacy, because he was 'out of line'. And what better way to silence him than simply to avoid and ignore him, first by not taking his classes, and then by not promoting him to the professorship he deserved on the merits of his thinking.

Dunham's inability to reach significant milestones in the academy is shadowed by the systemic racism he had to overcome, which includes the limited opportunities for African American scholars to publish their work. Not only were there "few opportunities for African Americans to enter the academy" (McClendon & Ferguson, 2019, p. 31), but "in some instances, the doctoral dissertation is the only available source for a clue into the philosophical views of Black philosophers" (p. 42). And when Black philosophers did find an outlet for their work, "the available academic journals were generally focused on disciplines outside of philosophy" (p. 42).

This indeed seems to be the case for Dunham's article "The Concept of Tension in Philosophy". Notwithstanding the interdisciplinary intent of the editors of *Psychiatry*, Dunham's article would typically belong in the pages of the American Journal of Philosophy (established in 1879) or of the Journal of the American Philosophical Association (first published in 1900), both of which would have been ideal outlets for a paper that was precisely focused on the leading philosophers of the time who were also Dunham's mentors: Dewey, Mead, and Whitehead. Instead, we can infer that Dunham was 'relegated' to publishing his work in *Psychiatry*, however much it may have been a success for the journal's inaugural issue and for Sullivan's intellectual purposes. Despite the level of promise he showed as a philosopher, Dunham never published any of his own work after this.

African American Philosophy

Racism sidelined Dunham's thought just as it did to many other brilliant African American philosophers. This common phenomenon makes the work of compilations, anthologies, and authoritative review studies such as McClendon and Ferguson's that much more difficult to put together (it took them 25 years to complete this initial step), but also that much more important. This author must rely heavily on their work for the simple and telling reason that it is literally "the first step in the recovery and reconstruction of an African

American philosophical canon" (p. 3), and one notes with sadness the very recent date of its publication, 2019. Without these archeological efforts, we "are left with the impression that African American philosophers in the academy have virtually disappeared [and that] nonacademic philosophy remained the limits of African American philosophical contributions" (pp. 30–31). If not for these efforts, we are in danger of confirming that philosophy "will continue to march under the banner of 'FOR WHITES ONLY'" (p. 2).

From the forgotten, the overlooked, the discriminated, from the scholars who made it "through the back door" (p. 7), McClendon and Ferguson successfully recover a substantive body of work, 'African-American philosophy'. They successfully put it 'on the map' as an essential component of any worthwhile history of philosophy. "African American philosophers have developed a formidable body of work about philosophy, particularly about how the Black experience is related to the 'big questions' …[resulting in] African American philosophy as a legitimate area of philosophy" (p. 4). What then is African American philosophy?

It cannot be simplistically reduced to a particular point of view or specific philosophy; that would be doing a disservice to the richness and complexity of the tradition. As the authors explain, "African American philosophy does not boil down to discovering a consensus. *African American philosophy is not a collective worldview or community with a shared epistemology, metaphysics, or philosophical vocabulary*" (2019, pp. 96–97, italics in the original). Indeed, African American philosophy can regroup widely opposing positions and philosophical perspectives. "African American philosophy is simply philosophy that engages the African American experience and condition rather than a case of representing a unitary philosophical perspective, which is shared by all or even most Black people" (p. 98). And indeed, McClendon and Ferguson cover the thoughts of many African American philosophers, often in opposition to their own positions. But there is a thread running through the thoughts of African American philosophers that doesn't so much *tie* as it *links* their thoughts into a recognizable and substantive body of work. "African American philosophy can embody the concrete content of Black material and intellectual culture. In other words, African American philosophy - in its particularity - *can achieve* metaphilosophical justification" (p. 85).

In this sense, philosophical investigations are embedded in the historical circumstances that gave rise to them. In establishing the intellectual foundations of African American philosophy, McClendon and Ferguson align themselves with Alain Locke: "all philosophies, it seems to me, are in ultimate derivations philosophies of life and not of abstract, disembodied 'objective' reality: products of time, place, and situation, and thus systems of timed history rather than timeless eternity" (1935, p. 313). In what ways do the "systems of timed history" establish the ground to "engage the African American experience and condition"?

McClendon and Ferguson explain how Du Bois, a contemporary of Dunham, framed this ground. "African American philosophers were faced with a dual professional imperative: on the one hand, they undertook work that would gain the scholarly approval of their white counterparts. On the other hand, these segregated philosophers had a commitment to address the philosophical issues confronting the African American community. This dual imperative, which Du Bois had framed as a double consciousness, remained a salient feature of the history of African American philosophers, up through the final decades of the twentieth century" (2019, p. 47). They explain that this "dual imperative" opposed the scholars' "commitment to address the philosophical issues confronting the African American community" to their need to "gain the scholarly approval of their white counterparts" (p. 47). This 'double consciousness' will be helpful in our attempt to situate Dunham not only as an American philosopher, but also as an African American philosopher.

In the thought-provoking title of his anthology of African American philosophers, *Philosophy Born of Struggle*, Harris (1983) clearly identifies the ground that gave birth to African American philosophy, and Du Bois sets the parameters of the challenge. Many took on the imperative identified by Du Bois in a straightforward way, by speaking forcefully to the black experience, and to relegate the imperative to gain white approval to a secondary position. As early as the 1880s, one of the most striking examples is Richard Greener, whose writings, disputing the image of white men raising Blacks up from degradation, stressed Blacks' roles in ending slavery and building their own freedom. This culminated in what Greener's biographer Katherine Chaddock (2017, p. 121) called "a large splash" in "his eloquent and creative approach to race relations". Greener redefined the 'problem' of race as "white bigotry" and not Black inferiority, leading to his groundbreaking article whose title coined the expression, "The White Problem" (Greener, 1894).

In Dunham's own time, the double imperative was becoming viewed as an either/or choice instead of an inevitable tension to be maintained. For instance, Paul Robeson forcefully argued that "every artist, every scientist, [every writer] must decide NOW where he stands. He has no alternative. There is no standing above the conflict on Olympian heights. There are no impartial observers. The battlefront is everywhere. There is no sheltered rear. ... He must elect to fight for freedom or slavery" (Robeson, 1978, pp. 118–119).

Robeson argued that it is the conditions of racism that force such a stark choice on all black intellectuals - either fight for freedom, or submit to slavery. So, for instance, McClendon and Ferguson believe, rightfully, that their work to put African American philosophy 'on the map' is part of that fight for freedom. But they recognize that they are far from their goal, and that "the continuing response of the philosophical guild to its [African American philosophy] presence confirms that its legitimacy is still not universally accepted" and in contrast to 'Greek', 'German', and even 'American' philosophy, "African American philosophy is seen as a semantic monstrosity bordering of self-contradiction" (2019 p. 5). This dismissiveness by the philosophical establishment is striking, but not unexpected. The label of 'American' philosophy suffices, the reasoning goes.

In this 'fight for freedom', McClendon and Ferguson show that African American philosophy has favored its own versions of 'imported' continental philosophy in order to find something 'beyond' its shackles, how could it not? "The African American turn to dialectical idealism was philosophically an affirmation of the principle of freedom" (2019, p. 16) and "a weapon in the fight against racism" (2019, p. 17). Over the course of the 20th century, the favored philosophical paradigm shifted to dialectical materialism, which is where these authors locate themselves. But, as pointed out above, African American philosophy cannot be restricted to any philosophical paradigm, and the authors cover how other paradigms have been put to use by African American philosophers.

One of these, more readily identified with American philosophy, pragmatism, is where one would most likely classify Dunham's thought. Indeed, not only were his professional relationships (Dewey and Locke among others) with renown pragmatists, but more importantly in his article, Dunham clearly identifies pragmatist philosophers as the sources of inspiration for the development of his thought.

As we situate Dunham's thought historically, we run into a deepening posthumous and tragic dismissiveness, coming from different directions. We have already seen how he was segregated and marginalized from the dominant philosophical establishment. But we can also note that he has been overlooked in two other important ways. His thought is in large part absent from African American retrospectives and historical anthologies; he is also absent from studies that have traced the philosophical origins of Sullivan's thought. Based on my research, Dunham receives biographical and bibliographical mentions, but his work is not mentioned in McClendon and Ferguson's review study and is similarly overlooked by such important anthologies as Harris' (1983) *Philosophy Born of Struggle* and Johnston's (1970) *Afro-American Philosophy: Selected Readings from Jupiter Hammon to Eugene C. Holmes*.

How might this be explained? Certainly his lack of published work is a factor. But given Dunham's status as a rising philosophical star, we might nevertheless expect that his dissertation (published as an article by Sullivan in contrast to many others' who were not that 'fortunate' to receive that degree of visibility) would be discussed as to its philosophical contents.

A probable, though by no means definitive, interpretation goes back to Du Bois' double consciousness, the double imperative. In some ways, it is possible to levy the criticism that Dunham does not fulfill the imperative to "address the issues that confront the African American", that he does not "elect to fight for freedom" and defaults to "slavery" in the words of Robeson. For instance, it is possible to claim that Dunham's 'pragmatism' leads to 'accommodation' to an unjust world. But this would be too narrow minded and dogmatic, since pragmatism can also be used to substantiate revolutionary claims. And, as we saw, the African American philosopher Locke, another pragmatist, is covered amply in these reviews and anthologies. But, in the case of Dunham, it is also possible to claim that the lack of any *explicit* statement in his article framing his thought within the discourse of the "fight for freedom" may suggest that he has succumbed to the pressure to seek approval from his white colleagues and mentors, and that he has abdicated the imperative to fight for freedom. The only other major publication Dunham participated in is a compilation of Mead's previously unpublished works at the time, which can be seen as paying homage to the white master.

In Du Bois' words, "we are bound by all sorts of customs that have come down as second hand soul clothes of white patrons", he concludes forcefully, "we can afford the Truth. White folk today cannot. As it is now we are handing everything over to a white jury. If a colored man wants to publish a book, he has got to get a white publisher and a white newspaper to say it is great; and then you and I say so" (1926, pp. 296–297). From this perspective, Dunham can be perceived as having been caught in "the race towards whiteness", as Langston Hughes coined it in the "Racial Mountain" (2002). Even amongst Dunham's contemporaries, from Du Bois to Robeson, this has been a daunting criticism, leading Franklin Frazier to reflect that "we have no philosophers who have dealt with these [philosophical] problems from the standpoint of the Negro's unique experience in the world" (1962, p. 32).

But it may be important to read in between the lines of Dunham's words, to see what may be implied, before taking the stance that the explicit absence of strong words to fight by means that the author's work is to be interpreted as an act of submission. By positioning himself in the seemingly apolitical domain of philosophy reserved for the dominant caste, by claiming this forbidden territory as his own, this may itself be seen as a subversive act. This is something that the students who dropped his class may have understood quite well.

In addition, turning our attention to the content of his thought, while he does not lay it out explicitly, the implications of his title, "The Concept of Tension in Philosophy", are hard to miss. Dunham does not just set about reviewing the concept across different philosophers; he in fact establishes the concept as ontologically foundational and central to human experience. And while he explicates the concept of tension within the frame of pragmatist thinking, it is clear that he sees tension as a struggle at the center of the human endeavor, both at the center of the psyche and of social relations, even if he does not use Marxist vocabulary to do so. He says, "the concept of tension has also been introduced successfully into the solution of problems in social and political psychological theory" (p. 90).

Even if Dunham's thought is not centered on the struggle of the African American experience, his philosophy is surely born of that struggle and speaks to it as well. Unfortunately, an elucidation of these connections exceeds the limits of this study. Certainly, any suggestion that his thought succumbed to the philosophical domain of the dominant caste (to borrow from Wilkerson, 2020) would be incomplete at best. This is not to say that the interpretation that he succumbed to the "race to whiteness", to use Langston Hughes expression, is false, but it is at least incomplete.

Dunham and Interpersonal Psychoanalysis

In situating Dunham's thought, we will now briefly turn to reviewers of the philosophical roots of Sullivan's thought. It is quite likely that addressing Dunham's thought, even if it was highlighted by Sullivan himself, simply did not register with these reviewers. They most likely would not have known that Dunham was black, and so it is not a conscious form of racism that is at play but precisely the kind of systemic racism that is frictionless, to the white person, but certainly not to Dunham. This kind of frictionless racism requires work, committed work, as Robin Diangelo so compellingly illustrates (2018). It would have taken a sustained commitment on the part of these reviewers to look into why it was that Sullivan credited Dunham, an unknown philosopher, with such an important intellectual role. But it was precisely because he was unrecognized by the philosophical establishment that he could so easily be overlooked, despite all the arrows that Sullivan points in his direction.

In addition to the journal's editorial note quoted above, in which Sullivan highlights Dunham's article as a most important and hence lengthy paper to help ground psychiatric concepts in philosophy, he then returns to it in *The Interpersonal Theory of Psychiatry*, this time singling out the article as crucial for bases of his own "system of thought". He singles out Dunham's article to "anyone who is interested in the philosophical justification of the concept of tension" (p. 35), a concept which, it merits repeating, is foundational for Sullivan's thinking. And, other than Lewin, Sullivan rarely, if ever, mentions any philosophical bases for his own thinking.

One would therefore expect Dunham to be mentioned in the studies that seek to identify the philosophical foundations of Sullivan's thinking. Not one! Perhaps the most striking omission is that of Cottrell's (1978) who, as a student of Mead himself, wrote an article in the pages of *Psychiatry* on the links between Sullivan and Mead. Not only is it ironic, and tragic, that the article appeared in *Psychiatry*, but let's not forget that Mead was one of Dunham's mentors and teachers. Indeed, the only other significant publication in which Dunham was involved concerned the editing of previously unpublished works by Mead (1938) - undoubtedly a work Cottrell had read.

Nor is Cottrell alone in this omission. Mullahy (1950), in a paper that links Sullivan's theory with the philosophy of Dewey, likewise ignores Dunham. Dewey, to reiterate, was one of Dunham's mentors and he figures prominently in Dunham's work. Thus we can see that the interconnections between Dunham, Dewey, and Sullivan are overlooked. More recently, Regan (1990) highlights the roots of Sullivan's thinking in his Whitehead's philosophy, but again without any acknowledgment of Dunham's influence on Sullivan. Finally, Green (1962), who accurately observed that "the impact of American philosophy definitely affected" Sullivan's thought, actually lists Dunham as one of those philosophers. While Green investigates the comparative links between Sullivan and American philosophers, Dunham gets no more than a listing in a footnote and no attention is paid to how Sullivan may have been influenced specifically by Dunham. The aim of this chapter is to redress, at least in a small way, some of these omissions. Before we explore the significant role of Dunham's philosophy in Sullivan's thought, it will be helpful to briefly examine Freud's relationship to philosophy in order to understand what Sullivan sought to differentiate himself from.

The Role of Philosophy in Psychoanalysis

Freud's attitude towards philosophy ranges from quasi-idealization to dismissiveness. This is well captured by Ernest Jones when he writes, "a reply Freud once made to my question of how much philosophy he had read. The answer was: 'Very little. As a young man I felt a strong attraction towards speculation and ruthlessly checked it'" (Jones, 1972, p. 32). On the surface, this suggests a personal ambivalence that explains the apparent contradictions between Freud's rejection of philosophy and his regular references to it. But Paul-Laurent Assoun (1976) suggests that this apparent ambivalence is actually part of a complex but coherent, even fixed, ideological perspective. Indeed, Freud's reply to Jones, describing the changes in his relationship to philosophy, capture what Freud sees as the change in philosophy's cultural position over the course of human evolution. As Freud explains, with respect to "the origins of our great cultural institutions—on religion, morality, justice and philosophy, ...psycho-analysis has established an intimate connection between these psychical achievements of individuals on the one hand and societies on the other by postulating one and the same dynamic source for both of them" (SE 13, 185).

According to Freud, culture's explanatory systems can be traced along an evolutionary/developmental arc from animism to religion, to philosophy, to science. On this developmental trajectory, philosophy falls somewhere in between religion and science, on one hand still retaining many of the primitive features of animism, but on the other hand striving forward towards science. "The philosophy of today has retained some essential features of the animistic mode of thought—the overvaluation of the magic of words and the belief that the real events in the world take the course which our thinking seeks to impose on them. It would seem, it is true, to be an animism without magical actions" (SE 22, pp. 165–166). Freud views the philosopher as the builder of large intellectual systems that are in the end mostly a narcissistic reflection of his/her own intellect, which explains its "strong attraction in his youth". The philosopher has the illusion of 'grasping' the world in his or her mind through this quasi-magical act, in similar fashion to an animist, for whom, as Freud puts it, the "idea rules" (p. 166), but it is also an attempt to incorporate the mature (secondary) process of reasoning into the apprehension of reality.

In Freud's system, the quintessential example of this narcissistic over-investment in the conscious mind is found in the construction of philosophical grand systems. Hence this philosophical fetishization of the conscious mind means that "the majority of philosophers will hear nothing of 'unconscious mental processes'" (SE 7, p. 266). Philosophy's refusal to adopt the notion of the unconscious can then be viewed as a resistance/defense to protect the philosopher's, or more generally philosophy's, narcissistic belief in its own "intellectual effigy" (Assoun, 1976, p. 84).

Embedded at the very core of philosophy, "there is for Freud a 'philosophism' that is practically synonymous with anti-psychoanalysis" (Assoun, 1976, p. 44), a narcissistic philosophism that Freud says he was attracted in his youth but had to 'ruthlessly check' in order to become a 'mature' scientist, a psychoanalyst. The mature Freud, better capable of delaying gratification, just like 'mature' modern Western civilization, is humbly and patiently guided by 'objective' science. "Psycho-analysis is not, like philosophies, ... seeking to grasp the whole universe. ... On the contrary, it keeps close to the facts in its field of study, seeks to solve the immediate problems of observation, gropes its way forward by the help of experience, is always incomplete and always ready to correct or modify its theories" (SE 18, p. 253).

While this kind of simplistic equation, philosophy = immaturity, and science = maturity, may elicit a smile or two today, Assoun makes the point that Freud's perspective should be seen in the light of German intellectual thought of the times when Hegel, in whom philosophical systemization achieved its apex in the early part of the 19th century, was being debunked, precisely by the challenge of science. Freud explains, "a *Weltanschauung* (equated with philosophy) is an intellectual construction which solves all the problems of our existence uniformly ... Believing in it one can feel secure in life, one can know what to strive for, and how one can deal most expediently with one's emotions and interests" (SE 22, p. 158). Philosophy is, in other words, "a narcissistic symptom" (SE 22, p. 59). But, just like a symptom, it is both a regressive movement back to the unconscious wish and a progressive movement towards its formulation, however distorted that expression may be. So, philosophy as symptom is then reconfigured as an intermediate stage between religion and science. In its progressive movement, philosophy comes back, returns, from its primitive sources in a transformed reincarnation, 'metapsychology', without which 'science' could not move forward.

We are now in a better position to understand Freud's response, as reported by Jones (1972, p. 32) - "Very little. As a young man I felt a strong attraction towards speculation and ruthlessly checked *it*". If by "it", Freud is referring to philosophy, then his rejection seems superficial and contradictory. But if the "it" is the "strong attraction", then we can understand how Freud believed he made available to himself, and to science, in a more dispassionate and objective way the true value of philosophical speculation.

Freud the scientist has to reach backwards in order to move forward. What Assoun calls a "speculative exigency" (1976, p. 65) is imposed by the brute facts, "in order to make sense of the facts themselves" (1976, p. 65). Freud introduces 'metapsychology' to refer to a kind of intellectual speculation 'in between' religion/animism and science. From this "intermediary position" (Assoun, 1976, p. 65), metapsychology can converse with both philosophy and science. At crucial moments, Freud explains, "we must use a bit of magic: the 'magic' of metapsychology in fact. Without metapsychological speculation and theorizing—I had almost said 'phantasy'—we shall not get a step further" (1937, p. 381). Its function is "to transform *metaphysics* into *metapsychology*" (SE 6, p. 259).

Metapsychology is a "mediating language" that "retranslates this [primitive] message, and delivers its true signification" (Assoun, 1976, p. 72). Like a dream (or a fantasy as Freud put it above), metapsychology is a regressive process that produces manifest content, and it is the job of the scientist then to analyze the speculative production in order to get to the psychic reality that remains unconscious. The work of dream interpretation can be thought of playing the same role as scientific explanation. Assoun (1976) tracks how Freud uses specific philosophical references in his argumentation. "Each time *he introduces one of the central psychoanalytic theses, one finds a legitimization through philosophical anticipation. In other words, for each fundamental thesis, Freud has the need to find in an eminent philosophical text a *precedent* (or several)" (p. 133). In this 'precise model', philosophy should be expected to anticipate scientific findings, and Freud the scientist should be expected to find in philosophy "a legitimizing and anticipatory echo" (p. 136) of psychoanalytic advances.

Freud admits, "I had therefore to be prepared—and I am so, gladly—to forgo all claims to priority in the many instances in which laborious psychoanalytic investigation can merely confirm the truths which the philosopher recognized by intuition" (SE 14, p. 16). Freud goes on to recognize that "the theory of repression is the corner-stone on which the whole structure of psycho-analysis rests" (SE 14, p. 16), and that it was anticipated by Schopenhauer, who was a particularly significant figure historically in the relationship between science and philosophy. Assoun quotes Schopenhauer, "the reciprocal independence of science and metaphysics is the guarantee of an ultimate unity, in which the 'gap' between the (metaphysical) results and experience is abolished" (p. 215) to show how his work in philosophy echoed Freud's in psychoanalysis. To illustrate, Assoun uses Schopenhauer's metaphor of two miners starting from faraway points who dig into the earth in their search, until the moment when "they see this upcoming and so anticipated moment of joy when each hears the pick of the other … It's as if Freud was following in reverse Schopenhauer's path. An echo, which in echoing the scientific word on the other side of the boundary, the scientific word echoed in philosophical speech, was filling it with substance, which in repeating it, accomplishes it" (p. 224).

While Freud's project for psychoanalysis is to emancipate itself from philosophy, psychoanalysis also relies on philosophy, through the mediation of metapsychology, for that very emancipation. We can appreciate how fraught, ambivalent, and yet 'precisely' theorized, this relationship was for Freud.

Freud's and Sullivan's attitudes towards philosophy are very different. On the surface, Sullivan's attitude is welcoming, in contrast to Freud's, as can be inferred by the inclusion of Dunham's paper as a central article of the inaugural issue of *Psychiatry*. However, other than footnoting the relevance of a philosophical work "to anyone who is deeply interested in [a] philosophical justification" (1953, p. 35 ff.), one is hard pressed to find any philosophical references in Sullivan's work, let alone as hinges in the formulation of his thought. So, for instance, when the rare philosophical reference is used, it is usually relegated to the status of a footnote (such as the above reference in which Dunham and Kurt Lewin are mentioned). In contrast, Freud's highly ambivalent attitude towards philosophy is explicitly unwelcoming, but he uses philosophy regularly to formulate his thought.

For Dunham, "one business of philosophy, as I conceive it, is to secularize, make available objectively, the flashes of insight and grounds of motivation that seem buried in the clouds of mysticism, religion, poetry" (p. 119), thus echoing Freud's positioning of metapsychology. We could then understand Dunham's article to be, at least in part, a philosophical formulation of 'tension' into a language accessible to science. Once "treated" by the philosopher, the sciences, and in particular the human sciences, such as psychology, psychiatry, and psychoanalysis, can then put the concept (such as tension) to speculative use for its own advances.

"The Concept of Tension in Philosophy", in Freud, and in Sullivan

Dunham Jr. organizes his study around the works of Alfred Whitehead, George Santayana, and Charles Pierce, in order to then formulate his thesis that the physical, biological, mental, and social worlds are foundationally interrelated in the concept of tension. At the same time, Dunham maintains the independence of each of these domains, resisting any reduction or appropriation of any one of these fields by any other. His position expresses the very purpose of *Psychiatry*.

Dunham starts with what he refers to as "basic" principles needed to think philosophically, even just to think, and one of these principles is that of "polarity", which can be summarized by the fact "that everything which exists depends for its being on the existence of what it is not" (p. 79). It is upon these principles that he then lays down the centrality of the concept of tension, which includes the dimension of temporality, which, when connected to polarity, gives us the dimension of the existence of what is being not yet. This is eventually translated into lived experience as the "experience of tension" (p. 79).

Dunham Jr. is attempting to establish a solid bridge of the mind and body split through the foundational concept of tension. "Whatever the metaphysical interpretation ... the concept of tension is neither mental nor physical exclusively. It is organic, which means that it is either or both. It constitutes, in a word, the conceptual passage from the 'physical' to the 'mental' or in the other direction" (p. 92). This allows Dunham to make tension foundational for all the sciences, from the natural sciences to the human sciences, to the social sciences, and of course, for psychoanalysis. "In physics, in logic, in psychology, the concept of tension has broadly analogous meanings" (p. 89). He goes on to explain that "tension is potential", which captures the futurity and the centrality of time, "it is 'historical' from the perspective of measurement but 'prospective' from the standpoint of potential energy" (p. 87). And this applies as much to physics as it does to psychology. He moves smoothly from the biological to the mental. Tension generates a "dialectical process" that "will proceed in a circle of perpetual tension and equilibrium" (p. 88); this process can then be applied to "the psychic organism [that] seeks to return to equilibrium; at the level of clear consciousness this becomes the urgency of desire; coupled with the initiation of activity it becomes volition". Hence, "psychic energy" (p. 89) follows a parallel process to physical and biological entities without being 'reduced' to them, and vice versa.

Accordingly, Dunham also applies this method of reasoning to "social and political psychological theory". As Dunham states: "The socialization of the individual can be viewed as a process of learning to control tensions, and to keep the proper balance between inner and outer stresses. The successful integration of the individual in society is the equilibration of the individual and society" (p. 90). Dunham Jr. elaborates on the foundational elements of the "experience" of tension to include "the pregnancy of the novel", "the potentiality for actuality", "the becoming of the organism" (p. 84), which, carried to the biological level and to higher mental domains, might translate into the term "appetition" that carries with it a felt "dynamic factor" seeking out "equilibrium" (p. 85) (though Dunham Jr. seems partial to Whitehead's more "colorful term, satisfaction"). Equilibrium then corresponds to the temporal phase of "completion" in the future, and disequilibrium to the present, but future directed moment of "incompletion" (p. 85).

Elaborating on time and change as intrinsic to tension, Dunham explains, "descriptively tensions are dynamic, directional, ambiguous - they are indices of events. ... As such they are presentiments of change, novelty, and emergence, harbingers of becoming. Their psychological history is a story in itself" (p. 92). Dunham is anticipating and countering potential charges of determinism, coming either from 'above' (such as psychic determinism) or 'below' (biological determinism'). Instead, he conceptualizes what he calls a "gradient effect". "The gradient is a dynamic tendency to react in a given direction if in a partially indeterminate one. The energy involved is no mythical stuff, but an integer the total gradient situation" (p. 97). He links this concept to Lewin and the notion of the total situation (field), and one can discern at least a dotted line to Sullivan's concept of the 'anxiety gradient'. In addition, change, and even more importantly the anticipation of change, are essential to Sullivan's distinction between the tension of needs and the tension of anxiety.

After taking on as a foil the philosopher's George Santayana's challenge to the fundamental aspect of change by introducing "changeless essences" (p. 101), Dunham effectively emphasizes the essential character of change, and tension. Having established the ontological nature of time, thingness, change, and tension, he is now equipped to take on the concept of relation, and of relation through language, the dialogic. "Relational analyses" then becomes a central dimension of the study of tensions, and specifically an understanding of the relation of "the subject to the other" (p. 111). And of course we cannot miss clear links to the concept of the 'interpersonal'. "We become aware of ourselves in becoming aware of the not-self" (p. 112), or, put simply, "self and not-self" as "self and other" (p. 112).

Dunham Jr. stays short of venturing into psychological and psychoanalytic waters, "the theory of the self is not to be deduced from polarity and relation" (p. 115). But it is clear that he distances himself from any philosophy that begins with the primacy of the 'I', conventionally attributed to Descartes. This will offer plenty of room to emphasize the foundational importance of the 'other'. Foundational, meaning not just that the other is complementary to the I but that the other lays the I's primary foundations. With the emergence of the 'other', the parallel movement in psychoanalysis, with the relational and interpersonal 'turns', cannot be missed. We can say that he laid the necessary philosophical foundation for Sullivan to initiate that turn.

As we saw earlier, Sullivan refers directly to Dunham's article as one of the philosophical sources for his own 'system of thought', and echoing Dunham, Sullivan explains that "in the realm of personality and culture, tensions may be considered to have two important aspects: that of tension as a potentiality for action for those transformations of energy; and that of a *felt* or wittingly noted state of being" (1953, p. 36). But Sullivan then goes a step further and classifies tensions into two significantly different types: tensions of needs and tensions of anxiety. In his explication of the tension of needs, Sullivan again echoes Dunham: as they are "transformed" into "activity", this calls upon the "neighboring future" so as to "remedy" the "disequilibration" of the being (1953, pp. 37–39). "The relaxation of the tensions called out by lacks of this kind I call *satisfaction* of the specific need which was concerned" (1953, p. 37). These passages read as though they were sourced from Dunham Jr.'s paper (though without being referenced as such). We will return to anxiety shortly.

This use of the concept of tension is common in psychology and psychoanalysis. We find comparable variants of it in Sullivan and in Freud; it will be how Sullivan then moves beyond it that will draw our attention. Freud's concept of tension, drawn from his reading of Ancient and Continental philosophy, is grounded in the human being's, the infant's, 'primary state'. "This primary state is conceived as a generator of tensions *(Spannungen)*, by which one should understand the state of lack that tends toward to be satisfied by escaping the insatisfaction that manifests simultaneously. This concept of tension allows the concept of need to take on an energetic and dynamic formulation" (Assoun, 1976, p. 93). Or, in Freud's words, "the principal function of the mental mechanism is to relieve the individual from the tensions created in him by his needs" (1913, SE 13, p. 186).

This is consistent with Dunham Jr.'s use of tension to link the physical, biological, and psychological domains. For Freud, tension is "a life principle", "a blind tension", "in other words, individual desire is nothing but the expression of the grand movement of tension, which, penetrating all the levels of the living process, comes to concretize itself within embryonic cells" (Assoun, 1976, p. 144–145).

For both Sullivan and Freud, the concepts of happiness and suffering are directly derived from the notion of tension. "What we call happiness in the strictest sense comes from the (preferably sudden) satisfaction of needs which have been dammed up to a high degree, and it is from its nature only possible as an episodic phenomenon" (Freud, SE 21, p. 76), bound to repeat interminably as Dunham laid out. And comparably for Sullivan, "the level of euphoria and the level of tension are in reciprocal relation", and "for my amusement ... may be expressed by saying that y is a function of x, and the relationship is y=1/x" (1953, p. 35). Up to this point, Freud and Sullivan are replicating the general philosophical consensus, but if we go back to Sullivan's foundational distinction between the tension of needs and the tension of anxiety, we will follow him on a radically new path that puts the 'other' in a position of primacy. Paradoxically, one can find fascinating parallels in European thinkers who, of all ironies, have claimed their affinity to Freud in their metapsychological formulations. Attempts in comparative psychoanalysis linking Sullivan to thinkers such as Lacan or Laplanche are rare, but offer a fruitful and challenging line of theoretical exploration, especially with reference to the concept of the tension of anxiety (Sauvayre & Hunyady, 2020).

Conclusion: Groundbreaking Steps

Seeking to make his mark on the intellectual landscape, Sullivan distanced himself from mainstream psychoanalysis. Beyond the different terminology, such as 'psychiatry' and 'interpersonal relations', a deeper and groundbreaking step can be traced to his concept of tension, in which he grounds a fundamentally different vision of the human drama. And this puts Dunham Jr.'s essay in a central position, not because Sullivan simply follows it, but because he uses to it move beyond it.

First, Sullivan introduces two radically different 'types' of tension in human experience, the tension of needs and the tension of anxiety. The tension of anxiety is radically different; indeed, "anxiety is a tension in opposition to the tensions of needs" (1953, p. 44) in a number of crucial ways.

Tension of needs can be met because there is a "remedy of the need" or a "satisfaction of the need" (1953, p. 38); there is the potential for the re-equilibration of the state of lack that the need is calling to be filled. Need can be identified, by the mother, and responded to through the identification and fulfillment of the need - he refers to this process as "tenderness" (1953, p. 40). In contrast, anxiety is not, and cannot be, remedied by the mother precisely because *"the mothering one induces anxiety in the infant"* (1953, italics in the original, p. 41). Further, "because of the absence of anything specific in anxiety, there is a consequent lack of differentiation in terms of the direction toward its relief by appropriate action" (1953, p. 42). Therefore, "anxiety is not manageable. It comes by induction from another person" (1953, p. 44). "This realm of anxiety [is] the easiest to overlook and the hardest to find" (1953, p. 44), and, at best, an anxiety 'gradient' can be established. Anxiety interferes with every healthy mental mechanism; "it can be said to cut off foresight" (1953, p. 44), both in the mother and in the infant, which is so crucial to the 'satisfaction' of needs. Indeed, anxiety "is in opposition to the tension of tenderness in the mothering one. It interferes with the infantile behavior sequences"..., "in fact, one may say flatly that anxiety opposes the satisfaction of needs" (1953, p. 44).

For Sullivan, anxiety functions as a foundational traumatic force. This raw or primal anxiety is not something that can be easily described, and while panic attacks may come close, they are still a far cry from this foundational trauma. Close cousins of this foundational anxiety include what Sullivan calls uncanny emotions such as awe, dread, horror, and loathing. At the core of the human drama, anxiety overrides needs. And he applies his unique understanding of anxiety to his entire system of thought, "insofar as you grasp the concept of anxiety as I shall be struggling to lay it before you, I believe you will be able to follow, with reasonable success, the rest of the system of psychiatry" (1953, p. 8). His 'system of psychiatry' includes his developmental scheme, his concepts of personifications, of interpersonal patterns (pathological and otherwise), of therapeutic action, and so forth.

So, the distinctive elements of anxiety in contrast to need are the following: it is induced by an 'other', it is not definable and knowable, its traumatic nature is foundational, and there is no such thing as a state of equilibrium nor satisfaction that eliminates anxiety, in contrast to need.

While need starts as a lack in the infant, and while it puts the (m) other on a crucial and equal footing in the search for a state of tenderness, anxiety puts the mother, as the originator and inducer of anxiety, in a position of primacy. This is a crucial 'turn' from an entire tradition that begins with the primacy of the 'subject' (from Descartes to Freud).

Arguably, this framing of core or primal anxiety in the other, and from the other, at the heart of the very (anxiety avoiding) structure of the human drama, is far more radical than most conventional 'two person' perspectives in psychoanalysis. All two person or relational perspectives emphasize the importance of the other, but not necessarily its primacy; that is, in Sullivan, the other can be considered to be the structuring starting point.

Even in a journal with explicit interdisciplinary aims, the inclusion, let alone the prominent position, of Dunham Jr.'s article, "The Concept of Tension in Philosophy", in the inaugural issue of *Psychiatry* is striking. It is striking, not really because it speaks to the progressive interdisciplinary nature of the journal, though to a certain extent it does, but rather because despite the explicitness of its prominence, it has been mostly, if not completely, overlooked in historical overviews of interpersonal psychoanalytic thought. In other words, Dunham Jr.'s thought is not just included in the inaugural issue of *Psychiatry* because it speaks to its interdisciplinary ambitions. It is argued here that Sullivan uses it to formulate the fundamental tenets of his interpersonalist system of thought. Sullivan clearly indicates that he has used Dunham's article as a springboard for his reflections on anxiety, which we can see are extensions, and even innovative reversal, of Dunham's formulations of the concept of tension. The fact that Dunham has been ignored given this central position is no doubt, to use Sullivan's own language, the sad result of 'selective inattention' meant to avoid the anxiety that underlies racism.

We can find here the primacy of the 'other' in all its forms, in theory and in practice.

Note

1. Biographical information is taken from McClendon & Ferguson, 2019.

References

Assoun, P.L. (1976) *Freud, la Philosophie, et les Philosophes. PUF*: Paris.

Chaddock, K.R. (2017) *Uncompromising Activist: Richard Greener.* JHU Press: Baltimore.

Cottrell, L.S. (1978) "Harry Stack Sullivan Colloquium: George Herbert Mead and Harry Stack Sullivan: An Unfinished Synthesis." *Psychiatry*, 41(2): 151–162.

DiAngelo, R. (2018) *White Fragility*. Beacon Press: Boston.

Du Bois, W.E.B. (1926) "Criteria for Negro Art." *The Crisis*, 32(6).

Dunham Jr., A. (1938) "The Concept of Tension in Philosophy." *Psychiatry: Journal of the Biology and the Pathology of Interpersonal Relations*, 1: 79–120.

Fontaine, W. (1983) "Social Determination in the Writings of Negro Scholars." in *Harris, L. Philosophy Born of Struggle: Anthology of Afro-American Philosophy from 1917*. Kendall/Hunt Publishing Company: Dubuque; pp. 88–106.

Frazier, F. (1962) "The Failure of the Negro Intellectual." *Negro Digest*, 11(4).

Freud, S. (1937) "Analysis Terminable and Interminable." *International Journal of Psychoanalysis*, 18: 373–405.

Freud, S. (1953–1974) *The Standard Edition of the Complete Psychological Works of Sigmund Freud*. J. Strachey, ed. Hogarth Press: London.

Friedman, L. (2014) *The Lives of Erich Fromm: Love's Prophet*. Columbia University Press: New York.

Green, M. (1962) "The Roots of Sullivan's Concept of Self." *Psychiatric Quarterly*, 36: 271–282.

Greener, R. (1894) "The White Problem." *Cleveland Gazette*, 12: #7. Ohio Center Historical Archives. http://dbs.ohiohistory.org/africanam/html/det347b.html?ID=18168

Harris, L. (1983) *Philosophy Born of Struggle: Anthology of Afro-American Philosophy from 1917*. Kendall/Hunt Publishing Company: Dubuque.

Harrison, E. & Harrison, F. (1999) *African-American Pioneers in Anthropology*. University of Illinois Press: Urbana.

Hughes, L. (2002) "The Negro Artist and the Racial Mountain." *The Collected Works of Langston Hughes*. University of Missouri Press: St. Louis.

Johnston, P. ed. (1970) *Afro-American Philosophies: Selected Readings from Jupiter Hammon to Eugene C. Holmes*. Montclair State College Press: Montclair, NJ.

Jones, E. (1972) *Sigmund Freud Life and Work, Volume One: The Young Freud 1856–1900*. The Hogarth Press: London.

Lacan, J. (1966) *Écrits*. Seuil: Paris.

Lacan, J. (1973) *Les Quatres Concepts Fondamentaux de la Psychanalyse*. Seuil: Paris.

Laplanche, J. (1987) *Problématiques V: Le Baquet*. PUF: Paris.

Laplanche, J. (2011) *Freud and the Sexual*. The Unconscious in Translation: New York, NY

Locke, A. (1935) "Values and Imperatives." In *American Philosophy: Today and Tomorrow*. S. Hook and H. Kallen, eds. Lee Furman: New York, NY.

McClendon III, J. & Ferguson II, S. (2019) *African American Philosophers and Philosophy*. Bloomsbury Publishing: New York.

Mead, G.H. (1938) *The Philosophy of the Act*. Charles W. Morris, John M. Brewster, Albert Millard Dunham and David L. Miller, eds. The University of Chicago Press: Chicago.

Mullahy, P. (1950) "A Philosophy of Personality." *Psychiatry*, 13(4): 417–437.

Regan, T. (1990) "The Matrix of Personality: A Whiteheadian Corroboration of Harry Stack Sullivan's Interpersonal Theory." *Process Studies*, 19(3): 189–198.

Robeson, P. (1978) "The Artist Must Take Sides." In *Paul Robeson Speaks: Writings, Speeches, Interviews, 1918–1974*. P. Foner, ed. Carol Publishing Group: Secaucus.

Sauvayre, P. & Hunyady, O. (2020) "Introduction to a Lacivanian Idiolect." In *The Unconscious: Contemporary Refractions in Psychoanalysis*. P. Sauvayre and D. Braucher, eds. Routledge: New York.

Sullivan, H.S. (1953) *The Interpersonal Theory of Psychiatry*. Norton: New York.

Wilkerson, I. (2020). *Caste: The Origin of Our Discontent*. New York: Random House.

Chapter 5

Reproduction and Resistance

Psychoanalysis in the Midst
of the Political Economy

Katharina Rothe

The interdisciplinary journal, *Psychiatry: Journal of the Biology and the Pathology of Interpersonal Relations*, first appeared in 1938 on the heels of the Great Depression. The time period was characterized by the effects of the economic crisis following the crash of the stock market in 1929 and an extreme socio-economic gap between social classes in the United States and Europe. In Germany, National Socialism was already raging, Jews and other persecuted people were emigrating to other countries, including the United States, and the Nazi regime was preparing for war. These events occurred against the background of the second industrial revolution, which had spurred the ongoing industrialization of Europe and the United States with the invention of the telephone, the building of electrical power networks, the construction and expansion of the railroad systems as well as of water and gas supply. Added to the progress of the natural and applied sciences was the emergence of such disciplines as psychology and sociology in the late 19th century. In the midst of these changes, Sigmund Freud invented the method of psychoanalysis in order to understand and alleviate mental suffering. As I will show in this chapter, psychoanalysis was interdisciplinary from the start.

In short, the psychosocial landscape held much suffering and faced the threat of fascism on the one hand, as well as the promise of immense scientific progress and hope for the betterment of human societies on the other. The first issue of the journal of *Psychiatry* reflects both of these sides and includes contributions from scholars in philosophy and the social sciences as well as clinicians from psychiatry and the psychological professions. The journal brings together

DOI: 10.4324/9781003270355-6

diverse scholars in order to tackle psychosocial issues that demand collaboration across academic disciplines.

I will take as my starting point two articles by Junius F. Brown (1938) and Kingsley Davis (1938) in order to rethink the interdisciplinary and political roots of (interpersonal) psychoanalysis. Brown was a social psychologist who combined field theory, psychoanalysis and Marxism. Davis, a sociologist, critically examined the implicit societal norms and values of the emerging field of "mental hygiene", which was both a "social movement" and an "applied science". I will discuss the stances each author takes in the context of the early debate between value-judgement and positivism in the social sciences in the 1930s, and I will link these debates to the dispute between the critical rationalists and the critical theorists of the Frankfurt School (originally known as the Institute for Social Research) that took place after 1945. Since the Frankfurt School broke with and polemicized against their former member, Erich Fromm, one of the founders of the interpersonal school, the demarcation of disciplines and compartmentalization that leave schools of thought boxed in and entrenched have persisted.

In the current sociopolitical context, it is inspiring to revisit the ways in which, over 80 years ago, practitioners and researchers in the humanities, the natural sciences and the social sciences joined forces to grapple with societal crises facing interpersonal and societal relations. But looking back can be disheartening because "the rising threat of fascism" that Brown speaks of was already raging in Germany as a result of National Socialism and would soon culminate in World War II and the Shoah. Today, fascism has become a renewed threat in the United States and Europe. At the same time, we are in the midst of a global pandemic that has exacerbated the immense economic disparity between a tiny minority of super-rich and the growing poverty and existential struggle of the vast majority. In other words, it is high time to reconsider the interdisciplinary roots of psychoanalysis, which will be the focus of this chapter.

Brown: Bringing Together Freud and Marx

Brown was born in Denver, Colorado, in 1902 and died in Beaumont, California, in 1970 (Stemberger, 2009; Stone & Lorenz, 1980). He was a student of Kurt Lewin, the German Jewish social psychologist, one of the Gestalt theorists and founder of field theory in experimental psychology. Brown contributed to teaching and studying gestalt theory at the Universities of Colorado and Kansas. His major social psychological work *Psychology and the Social Order* (1936) was amongst the most influential of American social psychology in the 1930s and 1940s. He combined field theory, psychoanalysis and Marxism. Because of his Marxism, he was isolated academically in the McCarthy era of the 1950s. He maintained a private practice as a psychotherapist through 1959.

His short essay of 1938, entitled "Freud vs. Marx: Real and Pseudo Problems Distinguished", has the character of a polemic rather than a scholarly article. Discussing Freudian versus Marxian theory, Brown juxtaposes the two theories as part of the disciplines of psychology and sociology; they stand out to him "in Appalachian eminence" against a field he otherwise devalues sharply as "the flat lands of social science" against the "Himalayas" and "Rockies" of the natural sciences (Brown, 1938, p. 249). He considers both as social sciences that had still "lagged behind" the natural sciences of the time. From today's perspective, Brown idealizes the natural sciences rather uncritically. While having made immense progress, be it in industrial production or in medicine, the natural sciences of the time also produced theories of the biological inferiority of 'the female sex' as well as eugenics and theories of different human races, including 'the Whites', 'the Negroes', and 'the Jewish' people.

Stating that his goal is "to win the fight for a stable social system", Brown explicitly advocates for a political stance that the two disciplines could achieve once "the truly scientific findings of Marx and Freud" (p. 249) would be separated from what he considers the non-scientific. The immense social problems of his historical time are the driving force towards the application of those theoretical systems, social and psychological "engineering" being the ultimate aim (p. 249). In Brown's framework, the field of social sciences reaches from biology to social philosophy, with the disciplines of "psychology, social psychology, sociology, and economics" lying in between. While Freud's "interests were pushed" from biology to psychology, those of Marx went from social philosophy to "sociological economics" (p. 250). The genius of both scholars, according to Brown, lay in each of their systematizations, one of "economic determinism" in the case of Marx, one of "psychological determinism" in the case of Freud (p. 250). But Freud spoke of "psychical", not psycho-logical determinism (Freud, 1901, p. 252), which might already be taken as a hint of the way Brown 'applies' Freudian theory.

Upholding the epistemology of the natural sciences, Brown considers "deduction" as the proper scientific method. He criticizes "a mere accumulation of statistical data" versus "systematic theory [...] which stringently attempts to deduce facts on the basis of certain first premises" (p. 250). One such Marxist 'first premise' is that "societal being determines consciousness", and not vice versa (Marcuse, 1958, p. 41; Marx, 1859). Yet, the author does not elaborate. Freudian science is summarized as the theory of the "psychosexual genesis" of neuroses (p. 251), and brief examples of "applied psychoanalysis" demonstrate that Brown refers to the application of bits of a psychoanalytic theory of personality in order to understand people's internal conflicts biographically, e.g., when he suggests it would be interesting to strengthen "the case against Trotsky" "by a little Freudian analysis" (p. 251). Although we might think of *a dynamic unconscious* as Freud's "first premise", Brown does not mention the word 'unconscious' in his brief 1938 article. By contrast, he does discuss the unconscious in other articles (Brown, 1937), in which he lays out how Kurt Lewin's topological and experimental psychology might be combined with psychoanalytic concepts.

Having studied with Lewin, Brown uses a typical tool of field theory by drawing a graph of a coordinate plane on which both Freudian and Marxist theoretical systems are represented by two sets of concentric ellipses with the center of the overlapping region being at the point of origin of the graph. Starting from the center of each ellipse, we find successively the respective "regions of scientific postulation", the "regions of legitimate implication", and that of "suggestive speculation". The region of scientific postulation of one system slightly overlaps with the region of suggestive speculation of the other. Commenting on dismissals of Freudians by Marxists, and vice versa, which were common in the 1930s, Brown calls those that stem from this overlap "meaningless problems" (Brown, 1938, p. 251). He basically states that Marxists didn't know enough of Freudian theory, and the same goes for Marxists about psychoanalysis. He mocks an imaginary Freudian who might "work trying to deduce [...] economic facts from libido theory" (p. 254). At the center of fruitful cooperation, however, Brown considers the overlapping region of "legitimate implications" of both theories; that is *social psychology*.

When Brown comes to speak about the region of social psychology, "overlapping of the legitimate implications of both theories", and hence "full of genuine problems", he briefly mentions the "problem of woman" (p. 254).[1] By "problem", he means the "disequality between the sexes" (p. 254), which, from a Marxian perspective, would not exist in a "classless society" (p. 255), whereas, from a Freudian perspective, there still would be a "special [...] feminine psychology" (p. 255). Without discussing the issue further, he simply claims that if the disequality of the sexes were to be understood through Marxism, it should be non-existent in the Soviet Union. According to his polemic, the same logic applies to the "problems" of "homosexuality and prostitution" (p. 255). Since all identified "problems" still existed, neither Freudianism nor Marxism could stand alone in examining the social-psychological field. As mentioned above, Brown is not simply concerned with the scientific investigation of the field; rather, in line with the overall aim of social-psychological studies, he proposes to solve psychosocial problems, to either change "human nature to fit the world of industrialized production" (p. 255) or change "the nature of human civilization to better fit basic human needs" (p. 255). In short, the author reaches the conclusion that only through dialectically opposing both psychoanalysis and Marxism could such a fruitful science come about. However, given the brevity of his analysis, is he unable to achieve any such synthesis and he remains wedded to a binary model that contrasts the different perspectives with one another.

Davis: Against Psychologism and Conformism

Kingsley Davis was born in Jones County, Texas, in 1908 and died in Stanford, California, in 1997 (Heer, 2005). He was an American sociologist and demographer. His 1938 article, "Mental Hygiene and the Class Structure", critically examines the implicit societal norms and values of the then emerging field of "mental hygiene", both as a social movement that was officially founded in 1908 and as an applied science. It will become apparent how this movement found its continuation in the contemporary field of mental health[2] (or behavioral health), and how it has come to be known as "managed care" in the language of the insurance industry.[3]

Davis builds on the work of Max Weber (1904-05), *The Protestant Ethic and the Spirit of Capitalism*, which was translated into English and introduced by Davis's teacher, the well-known sociologist Talcott Parsons, in 1930. Drawing on Weber, Davis demonstrates how the "vertical dimension in society" corresponds exactly "with the social" (Davis, 1938, p. 55). Its "crystallized hierarchy" was supported by a "system of sentiments and legal and moral sanctions" on one hand, plus "interpersonal relations" on the other hand (p. 55). Davis analyses "the mobile class system" and its "world philosophy" as characterized by the philosophy of an "open class society" (p. 55). Summarizing Weber's account of Protestant ethics, while also quoting his peer Robert Merton[4] on the same subject, Davis describes the "Protestant ethic" as:

1 "Democratic", as it was based on the idea of meritocracy versus aristocracy][5],
2 "Worldly", with the "accumulation of wealth" and "achievement of status" at its center,
3 "Ascetic", favoring sobriety and abstinence,
4 "Individualistic", "placing responsibility upon the individual",
5 "Rationalistic and Empirical in assuming a world order discoverable through sensory observation of nature" and
6 "Utilitarian in pursuing practical ends [...] conceiving human welfare in secularized terms as attainable by human knowledge and action".

With the field of "mental hygiene" having incorporated this "ethic not just consciously but unconsciously", it was therefore "susceptible to the psychologistic approach to human conduct" that "served to obscure the social determinants of mental disease" and especially "the effects of invidious or emulative relationships" (p. 56). The field was thus prone to lapse into being "preventive" because it didn't allow for the analysis of the "social elements", which the author sets out to identify (p. 56).

In other words, Davis critically examines the ideology of capitalism, where "vertical mobility [is] taken for granted", competition assumed, and — one could add — in fact 'naturalized' to this day as a Darwinian 'law of nature'. The implied rules of mental hygiene were 'to not envy' and to be "good sports" in order to prevent delinquency. "The healthy person is regarded as achieving victory [...] within the rules, by empirical-rational ingenuity and ascetic self-discipline". According to these rules, "[P]arents must not coddle" and make children unfit for competition and acknowledge the factors of "capacity" and "circumstance" (p. 57). In this normative and prescriptive set of values, "self-indulgence" is frowned upon, and "enjoyment", while not forbidden, should not make one "unfit for the serious business of life" (p. 58). According to Davis, the individual was seen through the lens of an entrepreneur. "Mental health" was regarded as the "satisfaction of individual needs", "desires, and mental processes", as if those were 'only natural', while ignoring how human nature should be considered as both social and biological. As such, a division of labor with implied "specialization" into different kinds of work based on different individual capacities was considered an essential aspect of Utilitarianism. As Davis states, "[T]o function, to grow, to do is regarded the purpose of life. Tangible ends and Progress are regarded as the goals. Human welfare is seen as attainable by the application of rational science" (p. 58).

The author goes on to discuss how those in positions of power in the United States at the time were predominantly members of the upper middle class, mostly of British descent, protestant and from New England. This white Anglo-Saxon protestant elite held a belief in "humanitarian individualism" (p. 58), based on the idea that initiative and striving, paired with abstinence, would lead to success. Failure would be attributed to the individual alone. Consequently, adjustment to the moral values of the upper middle class were equated with mental health. What would be considered "normal" was not a statistical average throughout the population, but rather an ideal, imbued with "ethical meaning" (p. 58), which was retroactively justified "on 'scientific' grounds" (p. 58).

Davis criticizes the "psychologistic conception of human nature" (p. 60), the "explanation of human conduct in terms of traits originating within the individual, as over against [...] originating within society". "[M]otives, drives, instincts, urges, prepotent reflexes", Davis explains, were conceptualized in a purely individualistic way while "ignoring the social genesis of what is called by these names" (p. 60).

The result of these "implicit assumptions" and the neglect of "social elements" as "determining factors" (p. 61) therefore leads to the conflation of conformity to the norms and values of the ruling class with "mental health" (p. 63). His sociological analysis, by contrast, considers the "individual's perception of his role in the eyes of others" as significant. The 'individual self' only developed "through the acquisition and internalization of the attitude of others" via "symbolic communication". Thus, for Davis, the "key to the relation between organism and culture lies [...] in the dynamics of the social role" (p. 63).

In short, Davis criticizes the psychologism and conformism of the field of mental hygiene from a sociological point of view, suggesting that "psychic conflicts inevitably result" from the "conflicting principles of social organization based on incompatible values.... [E]nds may be presented to one group as possible and desirable when in fact they are made impossible for that group by a conflicting mode of dominance" (p. 63). As an example, he refers to black people in the United States at the time of Jim Crow, segregation and unequal rights.

Finally, Davis defines a major ongoing dilemma for the "mental hygienists" in the terms of the period the paper was written, which we may easily translate to mental health professionals in contemporary terms:

> Scientific knowledge of mental disorder requires knowledge of social determinants. But there is a social restriction upon the impersonal analysis of personal relations, and especially upon the use of knowledge thus gained. [...] [S]uch knowledge must be employed only for culturally prescribed ends and persons who believe in these ends. Unfortunately, if one serves and believes these cultural ends, one cannot analyze social relations objectively.
>
> (Davis, 1938, p. 65)

If the "mental hygienist will continue to ignore the dilemma", he will "continue to be unconscious of his basic preconceptions at the same time that he keeps on professing objective knowledge" (p. 65). Davis thus concludes by formulating the core dilemma of social scientists — which can be easily extended to psychoanalysts — in that they attempt to analyze human relationships that they are inevitably deeply implicated in. Building on Weber's analysis, he shows how normative value-judgements stemming from protestant ethics and upper middle class whites in his historical era are inherent to the emerging field of "mental hygiene" that found its succession in the field of "mental health".

From today's perspective of a mental health professional, looking at the contemporary mental health field, we find that this dilemma is still widely ignored. The discipline of psychology still focuses on the individual and fails to see development deeply embedded in the social from the very beginning (that is, from birth or even intrauterine). Mental health is still equated with a mental organization that is adjusted to the dominant set of values, and it is still equated with 'functioning' according to these norms and values while they themselves remain unexamined; yet, they normatively determine what is 'normal', 'healthy' versus 'deviant' or 'pathological'. Whenever a mental health professional diagnoses and uses the systems of classification of mental illness and disorders, they also make implicit statements about which character-formations and behaviors are socially acceptable, regarded as 'well-adjusted' versus those that are not, and therefore have to be changed. Such practice is well maintained by an ideology that claims that psychology or the social sciences in general are free from value-judgments, just like the natural sciences.

Let us pause for a moment to examine if and how Davis' analysis of the field of mental hygiene is still relevant today, regardless of whether Protestantism is explicitly invoked, starting with the seven sets of protestant values quoted above: the idea of a democratic society built on meritocracy can still be considered a dominant value, so is the focus on the "worldly" "accumulation of wealth" and "achievement of status". This set of values is based on the idea that we get what we deserve: gaining wealth and thus achieving social status and power are basic functions of our economic system. Individualism is also still part of the dominant ideology and so are Rationalism, Empiricism and Utilitarianism. The idea of, and push for, evidence-based treatment methods that are supposed to make the individual functional or "effective" again (Selva, 2020) can be seen as derived from Rationalism, Empiricism and Utilitarianism. The definition of the Education Law of New York State for the professional practice of psychology also demonstrates these norms to be implicit in the field of mental health: "the observation, description, evaluation, interpretation, and modification of behavior for the purpose of preventing or eliminating symptomatic, *maladaptive* or undesired behavior; enhancing inter-personal relationships, personal, group or organizational effective-ness and work and/or life *adjustment*" (author's italics). The only one of the seven aspects on Davis' list that may not be explicitly part of the contemporary version of this ideology, norms and values is "asceti-cism". However, in my clinical experience, patients will still frown upon (self-)indulgence. While having the desire to 'be lazy' or 'indul-gent', patients will criticize themselves for these desires (see below). Instead, this falls in line with the values/ideas of the Protestant Ethic, according to which we have to work hard in this world in order to be redeemed as opposed to obtaining absolution through indulgences paid to the church (as was common practice in Europe before Martin Luther initiated the protestant revolution) (Rothe & Decker, 2019; Decker et al., 2013).

Clinical Examples of the Internalization of the Protestant Ethic in Self-Exploitation

In my clinical work, I frequently witness my patients' pressure to become 'perfect', which, per definition, is impossible. They are strongly identified with the norm to relentlessly work and 'optimize' themselves into ever more effective and productive entrepreneurs or employees. 'Buying into' the promise of redemption through pros-perity, they suffer from stress and a constant fear of failure. The logic under which they operate is based on the binaries of either/or, all/nothing, winner/loser.

One patient, for instance, is convinced that ostentatiously success-ful and powerful people 'have made it' because they work constantly. Symbols of wealth such as yachts, for her, translate into her vacation being "undeserved"; when she does not want to go to work, clean up her apartment or wash the dishes, she is being "lazy". Rich people, men, for instance, who own a yacht and sail around the Caribbean Sea, "deserved it, because they worked hard all the time", she says.

A patient, whose perfectionism I had pointed out a few times in ses-sions, suddenly has a revelation. "I was just gonna say: I'm not a perfec-tionist. I never manage to do something perfect!" She laughs, realizing that she'd thought a perfectionist was actually being perfect....

Another patient is also very strongly identified with working hard at all times at his own expense. Through suffering, he feels gratification, it's a sort of martyrdom that elevates him. Outside of his work, he goes to the gym where he frequents a group run by a very forceful trainer who makes the members feel like they are part of an elite club. The patient is very aware of the internal hierarchy and very keen on staying 'on top'. He is part of the "first row" of the group, which means, that he holds the power to actively keep people out or invite them into the in-group. He says, he "could make a ranking spreadsheet, but that would feel totally shitty"...

There also is a flip side to the 'rat race' of competition and perfectionism that goes along with the devaluation of whatever we compete over: as we will find in old fairy tales, where shit turns into gold/money and vice versa, one patient put it into the following phrase: "New York City is a place where millions of rats are competing over what really is a giant turd".

When the realization sets in that there is no winning the 'rat race', that one can never become 'perfect' or even good enough, envy and rage of what others are perceived or believed to have sets in. It might be expressed against those "up there", the rich and powerful, or the rage is displaced onto groups of 'others', namely minorities against whom authoritarian aggression can be expressed within a social consensus. This is where the social/cultural framework of racism comes into play, as a framework through which we can perceive the world and that we can use to channel aggression.

In the consulting room, this kind of envy and rage may be displaced onto minorities or, in the case of one patient, even onto animals. A patient talks about their not wanting to work their day job. While being strongly identified with the imperative to be productive at all times, they also feel resentful of having to work in order to make a living. They feel impinged upon by capitalism and envy their dogs, at some point bursting out in session: "Get the fuck away from me, I don't owe you anything". "They are entitled, just playing around all day and doing nothing". The patient is, as we understand from this outburst, envious of their dogs and, at the same time, of anyone who seems to make money without putting in much work. Therefore, we may also understand the outburst in the transference to the analyst, who seems to be making money just listening to her patients.

After my interpretation of this envy and rage, we get more into this form of impotent protest against capitalism. The patient is still very angry about having to work for money and says: "I want salvation to come and take me away from this job". When the analyst asks, "how? through god?", they respond saying, "well, definitely not through me, I don't want to do the work", and a little later "I don't want to negotiate with capitalism" but rather "be my own master".

A third variation of how people may react to the societal pressure described above is through the internalization of the aggression, i.e., the rage is being displaced against the patient's own self. Patients will 'beat themselves up', such as in: "I am pathetic", "I'm a failure", "I don't deserve anything good", or even, in a more extreme form, "I don't deserve to live". Yet, at the same time, patients who beat themselves up, metaphorically, or even literally, will often feel morally superior. When they employ a double standard towards themselves versus all others, they feel as if they achieve moral superiority by the harsh treatment of themselves. The masochistic 'pleasure' lies in the hidden grandiosity of treating themselves as if they were the greatest of all failures.

The Positivist Disputes in the Social Sciences

Since both Brown and Davis take implicit epistemological and methodological positions in what has become known as the 'Positivist Dispute' in German academic literature, I will discuss them in this context and then link it back to the question of the interdisciplinary position of psychoanalysis.

Both Brown and Davis align with Max Weber's critical stance against the positivist worldview and empiricist methods in the emerging social sciences. The first value judgment dispute in sociology was mainly about the question whether or not value judgments, which are inevitably part of social science, should directly determine social policy. Although often quoted as a proponent of value-free science — not the least due to the title of his paper "'Objectivity' in Social Science and Social Policy" (Weber, 1904), Weber argued that "[t]here is no absolutely objective scientific analysis of culture […] of 'social phenomena' independent of special and 'one-sided' viewpoints according to which expressly or tacitly, consciously or unconsciously they are selected, analyzed and organized for expository purposes" (p. 72).

Weber differentiated between means and ends; he did not deny that values are intrinsic to social science; on the contrary, he clarified how they can be found from the start in the very identification of what qualifies as meaningful problems and the formulation of research questions. "All knowledge of cultural reality, as may be seen, is always knowledge from *particular points of view*" (p. 81; italics in the original).

While Weber formulated a decisive stance against the claim of normative value-judgements to directly *determine* social policy, he nonetheless recognized them as inevitable in the social sciences. Thus, maintaining the separation between science and politics, he critically analyzed the implicit norms and values in the social sciences. Brown disagrees with that separation while holding on to a belief in deterministic sciences. He clearly upholds an explicit methodological position without discussing the underlying epistemology. By contrast, and just like Weber, Davis questions the very norms and values implicit in the field of mental hygiene.

This debate evolved into the 'Second Positivism Dispute' at the center of which are the Critical Theorists of the Frankfurt School who maintained that value-free social science was a myth in itself.[6] Even their opponent and critical rationalist, Karl Popper, admitted:

> It is [...] not just that objectivity and freedom from involvement with values ('value freedom') are unattainable in practice for the individual scientist, but rather that objectivity and freedom from such attachments are themselves values. And since value freedom itself is a value, the unconditional demand for freedom from any attachment to values is paradoxical.
>
> (Popper, 1976, p. 97)

Popper was quick to dismiss this argument as irrelevant and replaces the demand for freedom from attachment to all values by the demand that it should be one of the tasks of scientific criticism to point out confusions of value and to separate purely scientific value problems of truth, relevance, simplicity, and so forth, from extra-scientific problems (p. 97f).

While recognizing the problem, Popper holds on to a belief in the critical rationality of the scientist. This is essentially Brown's stance, who, like Popper, maintains a strong belief in rationality and *deduction* as the proper scientific method. By contrast, the Critical Theorists of the Frankfurt School highlighted the mythological, irrational underbelly in the seemingly rationalistic society, including the scientific methodology in the social sciences. As Max Horkheimer and Theodore Adorno state in the *Dialectic of Enlightenment*, "Enlightenment dissolves away the injustice of the old inequality of unmediated mastery, but at the same time perpetuates it in universal mediation [...]. It brings about the situation [...] which [...] constitutes one of the primal images of mythical violence: It amputates the incommensurable" (Horkheimer & Adorno, 1947, pp. 8–9).

It seems though that the proponents of Critical Theory were not above playing out this violence against each other, by excluding and polemicizing against one another, which brings us to the origins of psychoanalysis and to the 'mythical' violence that has pushed the interdisciplinary out of psychoanalysis.

The Interdisciplinary Origins of Psychoanalysis

Psychoanalysis originated from understanding and alleviating suffering; its roots have thus been interdisciplinary from the start. Freud developed psychoanalysis as a "science between the sciences" (Modell, 1984). Having started out as a neurologist and facing the limitations of medicine in treating hysteria, Freud ventured first into hypnosis and then invented the method of listening with evenly hovering[7] or "evenly-suspended attention" (Freud, 1912, p. 111) to the free associations (Freud, 1912, p. 116) of the patient.

Oscillating between neuroscience, medicine, philosophy, mythology and exegesis, Freud developed the psychoanalytic method as an interpretive, a hermeneutical one. He also explicitly made the case for interdisciplinary psychoanalysis and positioned himself against the American medicalization of psychoanalysis in his essay on lay analysis. In suggesting the idea of a psychoanalytic university, Freud writes:

alongside of depth-psychology, which would always remain the principal subject, there would be an introduction to biology, as much as possible of the science of sexual life, and familiarity

with the symptomatology of psychiatry. On the other hand, analytic instruction would include branches of knowledge which are
remote from medicine and which the doctor does not come across
in his practice: the history of civilization, mythology, the psychology of religion and the science of literature.

(Freud, 1926, p. 245)

We don't get to understand the psychosocial complexities of people's
suffering if we break it down to one side, the personal (bio- and psycho-logical) nor the socio-logical side (Davis), nor do we capture it
by the scientific method of deduction (Brown, Popper). Instead, the
psychoanalytic method invites us as practitioners to use our own sub-
jectivities — and that includes norms, values as well as affects and
our own unconscious — in order to analyze relational patterns. In
working with patients, it is through the transference relationship —
the unconscious transfer of relational patterns, or scenes, onto the
analyst — that we gain access to this layer of meaning.

Psychoanalysis has to 'hover' between disciplines because it is from
such a position that human suffering emerges, and it is in the cracks
that unconscious productions reveal themselves. For example, one
might think of slips of the tongues or breaks and contradictions in
our speech (Freud, 1901). The German psychoanalyst and sociologist,
Alfred Lorenzer, points out that "The misery that psychoanalysis
deals with both in therapy and in cultural analysis is as much 'internal' as it is 'social suffering'" (Lorenzer, 1986, transl. Rothe et al., in
print). Only from this in-between position can we analyze the histories of suffering:

> Let us remind ourselves that in the period of the origins of psy-
> choanalysis, without exception, people sought help from psycho-
> analysis, as they had become 'ill' from the pressure of dominant
> norms and values. Nothing has changed, insofar as the patho-
> genic pressure of societal conditions remains. However, the sit-
> uation has become aggravated in various ways, because the
> tension between individual desires and collective values has been
> distorted. Society's intrusion into the innermost core of human
> beings has led to a confusion of values. If the clientele of early
> psychoanalysis was mostly [...] the 'internally driven person', now

it is the *externally driven personality* that proves to be the task of psychoanalytic therapy. Repression has mostly given way to a *repressive desublimation*

(Lorenzer, 1986, transl. Rothe et al., in print)

It has been the project of Critical Theory to grasp the inextricable intertwinement of nature and society in the human subject. The Critical Theorists combined Marx with Freud to analyze the mechanisms through which the modern subject internalizes societal violence, and how power structures are internalized and reproduced. They explain that we have long entered an era in which coercion has become internalized to an extent that we enjoy (and suffer from) exploiting and commercializing ourselves — if we can — into ever more 'optimized' entrepreneurs and employees striving to consume and accumulate (as in the clinical examples above). Yet, even since the last economic crisis, the wealth gap has continued to grow significantly.

Forces Pushing Interdisciplinarity out of Institutions

In this last section, I will attempt to shed some light on some of the forces that pushed and kept interdisciplinary and critical psychoanalysis not only out of academia but also out of psychoanalytic institutes. Specifically, I will illuminate the violent side of imposing boundaries and fencing off others in the competition, for instance, by reducing psychoanalysis to medicine.

Firstly, the Nazis temporarily destroyed psychoanalysis in Europe by persecuting and murdering European Jews, amongst them many Jewish psychoanalysts. Freud was able to emigrate to London with his immediate family. Freud's decision to have James Strachey translate his works (with its emphasis on scientist and medicalized terminology) and to have Ernest Jones rescue psychoanalysis and become the "chief organizer of the psychoanalytical movement" (Roudinesco, 2016, p. 361) contributed to the medicalization of psychoanalysis in the United States. After World War II, psychoanalysis became part of the medical institutional mainstream in the United States. Traumatized through the Holocaust and in exile, many Jewish psychoanalytic immigrants seemed to be eager to assimilate to the dominant culture and medical establishment. As Kuriloff (2014) argues, the trauma of the Holocaust (having lost loved ones who were murdered, having been persecuted and having had to flee), as well as the often unac-knowledged fear that this might happen again, led Jewish émigré psy-choanalysts to conform with the medical mainstream in the United States in order to fit in. This situation was compounded by the fact that the American Psychoanalytic Association (APsaA) excluded all non-medical doctors until 1987, when the exclusion ended following a lawsuit (Mosher & Richards, 2005, p. 885).

This exclusion in turn contributed to the birth of interpersonal psychoanalysis, which, from the start had been interdisciplinary, as demonstrated here by the first volume of *Psychiatry* in 1938. Interpersonal psychoanalysts, including Erich Fromm and Harry Stack Sullivan, as two very different proponents, opposed main-stream, medicalized psychoanalysis in the United States. Another critic of ego-psychology and colleague of Fromm and Sullivan was Karen Horney. As Mosher and Richards point, any opposition to the mainstream held risks, and in 1941, Horney

> was demoted from training analyst to lecturer by a majority of those voting [...] at a meeting of the New York Psychoanalytic Society. After the vote was announced, Horney, Clara Thompson, and three younger members of the New York Psychoanalytic Society [...] walked out of the meeting and, later, resigned from the society (Hale, 1995, p. 143). The story, apocryphal perhaps, is that they stood outside the building on West 86th Street singing 'Let My People Go' and then walked to the bar at the Tip Toe Inn on Broadway, where they discussed founding a new Society. Later in 1941, Karen Horney and her associates founded the American Association for the Advancement of Psychoanalysis (AAAP).
>
> (Mosher & Richards, 2005, p. 870)

A further split occurred in 1943 when Horney sought to demote Fromm from her own organization. That same year, Sullivan, Fromm and Thompson joined with Frieda Fromm-Reichman, David Rioch and Janet Rioch to found the William Alanson White Institute of Psychiatry, Psychoanalysis and Psychology. Horney was not a part of the new institute.

In contrast to the medicalized mainstream of ego-psychology in the United States, interpersonal psychoanalysts emphasized the determinative role of culture and society in shaping the human being from birth. Opposing the ego-psychological understanding of the "instincts" as merely biological, the interpersonalists dropped the notion of the drive — mistranslated by Strachey as instinct — entirely. The Frankfurt School thus criticized and chased out their member Fromm and his fellow interpersonalist, Sullivan, for dropping Freudian drive theory. Adorno tarred them all with the same brush and called them "revisionist". He purported that precisely by sociologizing psychoanalysis and dropping the notion of the drive from psychoanalysis, they would take "the critical sting from psychoanalysis", because "natural human potentials never fully merge within the social order – especially in the given one" (Brunner & König, 2014, 491; Adorno, 1952, 1955).

At the same time, albeit in marginalized spaces, interdisciplinary psychoanalysis has also continued to brush up against the mainstream of the 'mental health' field. Yet, as is often the case in a competitive society, schools have been fighting each other over who holds "the truth" of psychoanalysis, rather than joining forces. As the sociologist Neil McLaughlin (1999, p. 112) points out, "Even though Fromm had an enormous influence on the radical and Marxist social science that emerged in the wake of the social movements of the 1960s, he largely dropped out of the canon of critical sociology. By the 1970s, Fromm was written out of the history of the Frankfurt School just as it was carving a small place for itself on the margins of the academy (Funk, 1982)".

The Frankfurt School's critique of Erich Fromm is an example of the way in which disciplines and schools of thought have become entrenched and compartmentalized. In a sense, competing schools have been reproducing and re-enacting the very societal economic and power relations that have shaped them, instead of analyzing and subverting them. Psychoanalysis has theorized the phenomenon of reenactment for a long time, beginning with Freud (1914) who contrasted unconscious repetition of conflictual psychic material to remembering; the term repetition has evolved into 're-enactments', particularly in relational and interpersonal thinking. What is being (re)-enacted unconsciously are relational patterns, be it in the consulting room or in the world.

Conclusion

I will conclude with the similarities and differences between the historical context of 80 years ago and today in relation to psychoanalysis and the social sciences. First and foremost, both are times of economic crisis, which have increased and exacerbated disparities between social classes and have been accompanied by a rising threat of fascism (not only) in the United States.

Then and now, both mental health and mental suffering are as much linked to social conditions as to familial, personal ones. In other words, they are psychosocial. However, the institutionalized field of mental health still separates the psyche from the social and fails to recognize the implicit biases and dilemmas concerning the practitioners' system of norms and values.

In the context of the United States, we might say that in spite of the Civil Rights Movement for racial equality, the increased emancipation of women as well as of sexual, gender and racial minorities, the ruling system of norms and values are still tightly linked to its roots analyzed in Weber's *The Protestant Ethic and the Spirit of Capitalism*. As Kingsley Davis highlighted, the proponents of this value system were protestant white Anglo-Saxon men of the upper class, the ones who benefit from and sustain the capitalist ideology and system most. With our contemporary society still being built on the wealth gap, and on wealth being passed on through generations and thus remaining even within the same families (Phillips, 2002), it is not surprising that we have also continued to internalize the fundamental norms and values still underlying our theories and practice of mental health.

We have thereby been reproducing and re-enacting the very societal economic and power relations at the very time that we have the methodological and theoretical potential and instruments to analyze them. American practitioners (clinicians and theorists alike) have been maintaining the divisions while being narcissistically invested in them. Competitive power struggles in combination with our "narcissism of minor differences" (Freud, 1917, p. 199) have exacerbated the theoretical differences between competing schools of thought. We have run the risk of losing the potential power of our interdisciplinary position.

Do we want to find ourselves largely swept up into the mental health field that is set up to turn suffering persons into 'well-adjusted', 'functional' individuals who will invest into marketing their/our "entrepreneurial selves" (Bröckling, 2015) or do we want to use our interdisciplinary and 'hovering' position to subvert and resist the mental health mainstream? To relate these questions back to this edited volume's theme of "breaking boundaries", boundaries can be important in that they protect, for instance, the safety and confidentiality of a patient in relation to the analyst. Breaking such boundaries would be destructive. Boundaries can also be set between disciplines, competing schools of thought and institutions. In the latter case, more often than not, what is being protected is not the integrity of a discipline or an institution, but they rather serve to exclude the competition (such as the competition of non-medical doctors in relation to medical doctors). Breaking or bridging such boundaries can free up potential for critical thinking. When it comes to the discipline of psychoanalysis, as has been argued here, it has found itself between several disciplines from its origins. The psychoanalytic method fosters the questioning and deconstructing of the status quo. This status quo is simultaneously personal and societal. Human suffering, 'pathological' relational patterns stem as much from the societal structure as from intimate family relationships. In the consulting room, such patterns are being partly repeated with the analyst, whose role is to help bring to light the origins of the suffering. As a result, the patient can be a little freer to choose how they want to deal with social and personal reality. On a larger scale, psychoanalytic thinking can subvert the status quo of the society, as it sets out to bring to light the irrational underbelly in our society. Yet, between schools of thought, we have all too often been fighting over the best, most precise, most critical psychoanalytic or psychosocial theory and practice, while the dominant political and economic forces have been running the show.

I would like to end this contribution by sharing my first association to the invitation to contribute to this book. In the year of 2009, Leipzig University, where I was working at the time, was celebrating the 600th anniversary of the institution. The motto read: "Aus Tradition Grenzen überschreiten", which translates to "A Tradition of Crossing borders". Amongst other aspects, the university celebrated famous former students and progressive moments of its history, such as having allowed as a guest in an auditorium the first woman.[8] I remember thinking how funny it was that the makers of the ad did not realize they might also evoke the German 'tradition' of crossing borders to invade other countries and thus having started two world wars. Reading this invitation rang both similarly and differently: it is the invitation to discuss and be creative with the foundation of interpersonal psychoanalysis as trans- or interdisciplinary. At the same time, breaking boundaries evokes associations to the violation of personal boundaries of another human, and, in the psychoanalytic world, of ethical boundaries in the relationship between psychoanalyst and patient. In this invitation, however, I read the pun as intended. It alludes to both sides of that which the breaking of boundaries can imply: a critical, fruitful, creative, resistant or subversive side — in this case of breaking academic disciplinary and institutional boundaries — and a violent side. In this contribution, I spoke to both sides and showed how intimately linked they can be to one another.

In short, I showed that psychoanalysis was positioned between disciplines from the beginning. Yet, what followed was the exclusionary fragmentation of schools of thought and of the disciplines in academia as well as in the area of practice. I interpret those as reproductions or re-enactments of the overarching capitalist power system. This goes hand in hand with psychoanalysis losing — to a great extent — its subversive potential of the interdisciplinary, which is what the 1938 volume points to.

Notes

1. This formulation evokes the similar one of "the Jewish Question" (see Marx, 1844). Today, we would consider these two areas as persisting problems of sexism and anti-Semitism, which have been discussed as interrelated in their modern form (Gilman, 1993).
2. The term "mental hygiene" is still in use as, for example, in the The New York City Department of Health and Mental Hygiene (DOHMH) (https://www1.nyc.gov/site/doh/about/contact-doh.page).
3. https://www.aetna.com/health-care-professionals/patient-care-programs/primary-care-behavioral-health.html.
4. Kingsley Davis was a contemporary of Robert Merton (who is famous for the notion of the "self-fulfilling prophecy" (...) at Harvard University, and both were students of Talcott Parsons, a "functional structurist" (...).
5. It does not become clear to me how meritocracy would necessarily go hand in hand with democracy. While Weber demonstrates a meritocratic belief system underlying capitalism, as a German sociologist in the

Kaiserreich, he only discusses democracy in relation to the Anglo-Saxon capitalistic democracies.

6. The Frankfurt School was a group of scholars at the *Institute for Social Research* in Frankfurt, namely Max Horkheimer, Theodor W. Adorno, Herbert Marcuse, Erich Fromm, Leo Löwenthal, Franz Neumann, Otto Kirchheimer, Friedrich Pollock and Walter Benjamin. They founded Critical Theory combining Hegel, Marx and Freud (https://en.wikipedia.org/wiki/Frankfurt_School).

7. Evenly hovering would be a literal translation of Freud's original German term of "gleichschwebende Aufmerksamkeit".

8. http://www.perfectforroquefortcheese.org/2019/12/aus-tradition-grenzen-uberschreiten.html.

References

Adorno, T. W. (1952). Die revidierte Psychoanalyse. In: *Gesammelte Schriften*, Vol. 8. Frankfurt: Suhrkamp, pp. 20–41.

Adorno, T. W. (1955) [1967]. Sociology and Psychology. *New Left Review*, 46, 67–80.

Bröckling, U. (2015). *The Entrepreneurial Self: Fabricating a New Type of Subject*. London: Sage Publications.

Brown, J. F. (1937). Psychoanalysis, Topological Psychology and Experimental Psychopathology. *Psychoanalytic Quarterly*, 6, 227–237.

Brown, J. F. (1938). Freud vs. Marx: Real and Pseudo Problems Distinguished. *Psychiatry: Journal of the Biology and the Pathology of Interpersonal Relations*, 1, 249–255.

Brunner, M. & König, J. (2014). Drive, Overview. In: Thomas Teo (ed.) *Encyclopedia of Critical Psychology*. New York: Springer, pp. 487–492.

Davis, K. (1938). Mental Hygiene and the Class Structure. *Psychiatry: Journal of the Biology and the Pathology of Interpersonal Relations*, 1, 55–65.

Decker, O., Rothe, K., Weißmann, M., Kiess, J. & Brähler, E. (2013). Economic Prosperity as "Narcissistic Filling": A Missing Link between Political Attitudes and Right-wing Authoritarianism. *Conflict & Violence*, 7 (1), 135–149.

Freud, S. (1901). *The Psychopathology of Everyday Life. Standard Edition*, Vol. 6, p. vii-296.

Freud, S. (1912). *Recommendations to Physicians Practising Psycho-Analysis. The Standard Edition of the Complete Psychological Works of Sigmund Freud*, Volume XII (1911–1913): The Case of Schreber, Papers on Technique and Other Works, pp. 109–120.

Freud, S. (1914). *Remembering, Repeating and Working-Through. Standard Edition*, Vol. 12, pp. 147–156.

Freud, S. (1917). *The Taboo of Virginity. Standard Edition*, Vol. 11, pp. 191–208.

Gilman, S. L. (1993). *Freud, Race, and Gender*. Princeton, NJ: Princeton University Press.

Hale, N. G. (1995). *The Rise and Crisis of Psychoanalysis in the United States: Freud and the Freudians*, 1917–1985. New York: Oxford University Press.

Heer, D. (2005). *Kingley Davis: A Biography and Selections from His Writings*. Piscataway, NJ: Transaction Publishers.

Horkheimer, M. & Adorno, Th. W. (1947) [2002]. *Dialectic of Enlightenment: Philosophical Fragments*. G. Schmidt-Noerr (ed.), translated by E. Jephcott. Stanford: Stanford University Press.

Kuriloff, E. (2014). *Contemporary Psychoanalysis and the Legacy of the Third Reich*. New York: Routledge.

Lorenzer, A. (1986) [in print]. In-depth Hermeneutical Cultural Analysis. In: Rothe, K., Rosengart, D. & Krüger, S. (Eds.). *Cultural Analysis Now!* New York: Unconscious in Translation.

Marcuse, H. (1958). *Soviet Marxism. A Critical Analysis*. New York: Columbia University Press.

Marx, K. (1859). *Zur Kritik der politischen Ökonomie. Marx-Engels-Werke* Vol 13, p. 9.

McLaughlin, N. (1999). Origin Myths in the Social Sciences: Fromm, the Frankfurt School and the Emergence of Critical Theory. *The Canadian Journal of Sociology/Cahiers canadiens de sociologie*, 24 (1), 109–139.

Modell, A. (1984). *Psychoanalysis in a New Context*. New York: International University Press.

Mosher, P. W. & Richards, A. R. (2005). The History of Membership and Certification in the APsaA: Old Demons, *New Debates. Psychoanalytic Review*, 92 (6), 865–894.

Phillips, K. (2002). *Wealth and Democracy: A Political History of the American Rich*. New York: Broadway Books.

Popper, K. (1976). The Logic of the Social Sciences. In: Adorno et al. *The Positivist Dispute in German Sociology*. Translated by G. Ady & D. Frisby. London: Heinemann, pp. 87–104.

Rothe, K. & Decker, O. (2019). (The Failing of) the Promise of Prosperity and Economic Growth as 'Narcissistic Filling' and Right-Wing-Authoritarianism. *Talk at the Association for the Psychoanalysis of Culture & Society (APCS) Annual Conference Displacement: Precarity & Community at Rutgers University*, 10/25-26/2019. In preparation for publication.

Roudinesco, E. (2016). *Freud. In his Time and Ours*. Translated by C. Porter. Cambridge, MA: Harvard University Press.

Selva, J. (2020). What is Evidence-Based Therapy: 3 EBT Interventions. https://positivepsychology.com/evidence-based-therapy (retrieved 9/10/20).

Stemberger, G. (2009). Junius F. Brown (1902–1970): Radikaler Feldtheore-
tiker – Brückenbauer zwischen Gestaltpsychologie, Psychoanalyse und
marxistischer Gesellschaftstheorie. *Phänomenal: Zeitschrift für Gestalt-
theoretische Psychotherapie*, 1, 38–41.

Stone, W. F. & Lorenz, J. F. (1980). The Social Psychology of J. F. Brown:
Radical Field Theory. *The Journal of Mind and Behavior*, 1, 73–84.

Weber, M. (1904) [1949]. 'Objectivity' in Social Science and Social Policy".
In: *The Methodology of the Social Sciences. Translated and edited E. Shils
and H. Finch.* Glencoe: The Free Press, pp. 49–112.

Weber, M. (1904–05) [1930]. *The Protestant Ethic and the Spirit of Capitalism.*
Translated by T. Parsons. New York: Routledge.

Chapter 6

Do *Less* Harm

Notes on Clinical Practice in the Age of Criminal Justice Reform

Julian Adler and Olivia Dana[1]

Surreal as it may seem, criminal justice reform in the United States has emerged as a veritable bipartisan issue. To illustrate, a recent article in *The Christian Science Monitor* announced the launch of a national criminal justice organization that will convene "Democratic and Republican governors, a Black Lives Matter organizer, and a Koch Industries vice president in an unlikely collaboration" (Thompson & Beam, 2019). Of course, this bipartisan support is typically limited to particular aspects of justice reform rather than a more muscular project of ending mass incarceration. For example, it often exists for a mode of reform that substitutes the provision of mandated behavioral health treatment (e.g., mental health and drug treatment) for traditional punishment (i.e., jail, prison, fines). With the opening of the first drug court in Miami-Dade County, Florida in 1989, and the subsequent rise of specialized courts and diversion programs throughout the country, an increasing number of clinicians are being hired to provide therapeutic interventions in criminal justice settings. And while the concept that therapeutic interventions are appropriate and humane alternatives to traditional punishment predates the current political and cultural recognition of a crisis of mass incarceration (e.g., this chapter responds to an account of court-mandated treatment from 1938), the current scope and scale of clinical practice across the criminal justice landscape is unprecedented (Marlowe, Hardin, & Fox, 2016).

As laudable as this may be, the criminal legal system can be a distinctly challenging—if not downright confounding—environment for clinicians; at nearly every turn, it requires a great deal of

DOI: 10.4324/9781003270355-7

conceptual and technical flexibility. Replete with complex treatment considerations, ethical dilemmas, interdisciplinary tensions, and a host of environmental obstacles, even the most accomplished practitioners will struggle to find their balance. This is especially true when the justice system has engaged clinicians in providing alternatives to incarceration. In these cases, clinicians must confront conflicting obligations—an ethical duty to their clients versus an institutional responsibility to the state, whose actors (judges, prosecutors, probation officials, etc.) expect accountability and accurate reporting about failures and missteps in treatment, which can result in courts taking punitive actions that can include incarceration. By any account, this is a precarious context for the formation and maintenance of a therapeutic relationship.

Beyond compliance monitoring, legal stakeholders may also have unreasonable expectations about therapeutic intervention as a "quick fix" or a panacea. The stakes in this struggle could not be higher: a robust therapeutic relationship *and* stakeholder trust are the cornerstones of effective practice across the spectrum of justice system roles and settings—and they can often determine whether an individual is confined to a jail or a prison cell or engaged and thriving in a community-based setting. Judges and prosecutors are also often the gatekeepers to treatment as an alternative to incarceration—meaning that lawyers, not clinicians, ultimately decide who can safely remain in the community to receive what they believe to be meaningful treatment interventions and who cannot. Casting aspersions on courts that offer drug treatment as an alternative to incarceration, one judge warns of "a dangerous psycho-judicial branch populated by judges who think they are doctors, who think drug addiction is a treatable disease, and who send their patients to prison when they fail to respond to treatment" (Hoffman, 2001, p. 172).

Reminiscent of philosopher Michel Foucault's (1977) seminal insight that the prison itself was initially conceived as a great humanitarian accomplishment (when juxtaposed with public torture, that is), some critics go so far as to argue that *any* clinical practice in the criminal justice context is inherently harmful. Notably, prison abolitionists contend that the criminal legal system in the United States is in fact so fundamentally broken that any attempt to reform its operations only proliferates harmful "forms of carceral control"—even bona

164 Julian Adler and Olivia Dana

fide therapeutic endeavors. "From New York City to Los Angeles, and across rural America, jail expansion has been chugging along largely because law enforcement continues to absorb social welfare work—mental and physical health, education, family unification," observe CUNY Graduate Center professor and renowned prison abolitionist Ruth Wilson Gilmore and James Kilgore (2019) of Media Justice. "To imagine a world without prisons and jails is to imagine a world in which social welfare is a right, not a luxury" (Gilmore & Kilgore, 2019).

As our title suggests, this chapter accepts the premise that even the most thoughtful and effectively-executed clinical interventions may retain some of the carceral taint of the surrounding system. At the same time, we affirm that clinicians have the potential to practice in ways that can reduce the overall harm wrought by the criminal legal system. "By drawing on psychoanalysis's rich account of the mind, with all its complexity and paradoxes, we have the opportunity to reform legal doctrine," argues University of Connecticut law professor Anne C. Dailey (2017, p. 14) in a recent effort to resurrect the law and psychoanalysis movement of the 1960s. Taking aim at the foundational legal myth of the objective, rational actor, Dailey envisages psychoanalytic ideas as conduits to "a more humane, psychologically informed, and fundamentally fair system of justice" (p. 14). Ultimately, this chapter does not seek to refute Dailey's claim as much as it seeks to temper it; we caution that the psychoanalytic sensibility has the potential to cut the other way.

Specifically, through a close reading of Ralph M. Crowley's "The Courts and Psychiatry" (1935), this chapter underscores the risk that clinicians may in fact lend further credence to biases enshrined in the criminal law (in Crowley's case, homophobia)—extending from courtrooms deep into the confines of consulting rooms. Far from self-executing and liberatory, this chapter contends that the intersection of psychoanalysis and the law may be a site where normative boundaries are more easily reinforced than broken. This may also have implications for potentially blinkered, unidirectional interpretations of countertransference in clinical practice, more broadly. By way of conclusion, the chapter points to a potential paradigm shift toward an ecological perspective that could serve to both mitigate this risk of bias and better align clinical practice with the project of humanizing the American justice system.

Crowley in Historical Context

In June of 2019, the American Psychoanalytic Association (2019, "Overdue Apology to LGBTQ Community") issued a formal, "overdue" apology for "past views that pathologized homosexuality and transgender identities." Inspired by the 50th anniversary of the Stonewall uprising in New York City, its press release acknowledged the role played by "the American psychoanalytic establishment" in perpetuating "discrimination and trauma." A case in point, Crowley's 1938 article clearly illustrates a direct nexus between this homophobic clinical bias and the operations of the justice system. The article describes his court-mandated treatment of Mr. Z, who was arrested on the charge of violating a sodomy law. Drawing an analogy to tuberculosis, Crowley opines that spitting in street "is an expression of pathology in the lungs, just as 'perverse' sexual acts are expressions of psychopathology" (Crowley, 1938, p. 266). "With most of *them* [emphasis added]," Crowley explains, "their sexual acts are the result of a 'compulsive habit' rather than real desire" (p. 268). Not surprisingly, Crowley joins the presiding judge in the view that "restor[ing] the offender to a useful place in society" (p. 266) ultimately entails "find[ing] a satisfactory source of love and affection in his wife" (p. 268). Mr. Z's court-mandated treatment is thus an alternative to incarceration that is predicated on the clinical pathologizing of his homosexuality. He avoids jail because he has a "sickness" for which there is a targeted treatment (conversion therapy, which is now understood to be a deeply harmful and offensive practice) that Crowley is eager to provide. For Crowley, treatment is a success when "for the first time in nine or ten years [Mr. Z] found that he wished to have intercourse with his wife. Marital relationships were resumed with much success. He was 'as excited as a bridegroom'" (p. 267). Moreover, Crowley reports that it was "a reassurance to [Mr. Z] that he wasn't really 'homosexual'" (p. 267). The scheme depends on the belief that a cure exists and that Crowley has got it.

At first blush, some readers might be tempted to rationalize our hindsight as 20/20 and defend Crowley's views as products of his time. Prior to 1963, for example, every state had sodomy laws on the books (Cavendish, 2010, p. 825). In the 1950s, all but two went so far as to classify sodomy as a felony (meaning the maximum penalty was a year or more in prison) (D'Emilio, 1983, p. 14). Penalties for first offenses ranged from a $500 fine in New York to a *life sentence* in Nevada (Manuscripts and Archives Division, The New York Public Library, 1964). Until the United States Supreme Court finally struck them down as unconstitutional in the 2003 case of *Lawrence v. Texas*, sodomy laws remained active in 13 states (Canaday, 2008).

Indeed, Crowley (1938) incorporates the very illegality of "'[h]omosexual acts'" into a tautological conceptualization of their pathology. "[M]otivated by resentments," Crowley argues that "[t]hey show their destructive character first in the fact that they are against the law" (p. 268). Writing from Rockville, Maryland in 1938 [Crowley later moved to New York City in 1946 to join the faculty at the William Alanson White Institute (Waggoner, 1984)], he might have had some sense that there were over 60 sodomy arrests in Baltimore that same year (another nine in Washington, D.C. and a sizeable 186 up the road in New York City) (Eskridge Jr., 1997).

Notably, this tautological mode of diagnosis was not uncommon. Writing in 1948, Irving A. Lanzer, who taught criminology, juvenile delinquency, and social work at the City College of New York, observed that mid-20th-century forensic psychiatrists similarly "[used] criminality to diagnose psychopathy and use[d] a diagnosis of psychopathy to explain criminality, even though there [was] no other evidence" (Lanzer, 1948, p. 29). According to Benjamin Karpman, professor and Head of Psychiatry at Howard University College of Medicine from 1921 to 1941, the reason why homosexuality and psychopathy were "often put together [was] because, in common with the rest of descriptive psychiatry, homosexuality [was] regarded as an antisocial behavior; *hence, by the same token*, as psychopathic" (p. 29). Tellingly, though, Lanzer criticizes Karpman for calling for the decriminalization of homosexuality because doing so ignored prevailing social norms and would cause the psychiatry profession to "[risk] serious consequences to its being and future" (p. 42).

Upon closer examination, however, it is critical to note that these prevailing social norms in 1938 were far from monolithic. Strikingly, Crowley even acknowledges that "[t]he notion that our present laws regarding sexual crime are archaic and unsatisfactory is *frequently* [emphasis added] expressed" (p. 265). He quickly counters that "the law is a reflection of prevailing attitudes," abdicating responsibility to the prospect of eventual "remedial legislative action" (p. 265). The point here is that Crowley is less a passive or unwitting product of his time and more a partisan proponent of the status quo. Buttressed by psychoanalytic ideas, he makes an affirmative decision to reinforce normative boundaries, i.e., pathologize homosexuality and perpetuate homophobia in the courts, rather than challenge them. Ostensibly, Crowley simultaneously avoids the need to question his own theoretical orientation in the face of growing opposition to sexual conservatism and its attendant oppressive mechanisms.

Admittedly, Crowley's flawed attempt at criminal justice reform can be further situated in the system's long and inconsistent (i.e., deeply ambivalent) history of attempting to rehabilitate—rather than punish—people in the first instance. University of Michigan Law School professor Francis A. Allen observed a "rehabilitative ideal" in American criminal law, which is "the notion that the sanctions of the criminal law should or must be employed to achieve fundamental changes in the characters, personalities, and attitudes of convicted offenders, not only in the interest of social defense, but also in the interests of the well-being of the offender himself" (Allen, 1978, p. 148). In other words, a "deviance"-causing illness that can be treated ought to be treated rather than merely punished. This rehabilitative ideal, which Crowley seemingly subscribed to, was the driving philosophy of criminal justice from the 19th century until the early 1970s, when it eroded under a sea change of public opinion and subsequent policy-making that reflected an increasingly punitive posture toward criminal behavior.

The 1970s was marked by efforts to stem rising substance use in American urban areas, and the War on Drugs catalyzed an increase in arrests and sentencing both at the state and federal levels. This shift in policy was characterized both by more aggressive policing practices and by sentencing reform that resulted in longer prison sentences for drug possession and distribution (Pearl, 2018). Rather than a justice system "grounded in faith of psychiatry and science" (Vitiello, 2013, p. 1276), the "tough on crime" reforms of the 1980s and 1990s were driven by faith in the deterrent effects of enforcement and incarceration. It was not until the late 1980s that the American criminal legal system saw a revival of the rehabilitative ideal—first through new treatment courts aimed at addressing drug addiction, then through the addition of "problem-solving courts" designed to address a variety of needs and populations through mandated interventions rather than incarceration (American University & Bureau of Justice Assistance, 2008). Modern-day courts are rife with clinicians who purport to treat the underlying drivers of criminal behaviors and judges who mandate defendants to their care. The slow and cyclical churn of the criminal legal system continues to move imperfectly toward more rehabilitative approaches.

Crowley in Contemporary Context

Regardless of whether Crowley is viewed as a product of his time, the more pressing—and unsettling—question is whether Crowley could conceivably be a product of our own. Homophobia persists in both clinical and legal contexts. Writing in *The New York Times* as recently as 1998, for example, journalist Erica Goode reflects that "[e]ven a decade ago, an admission of homosexuality by a senior analyst often meant a damaged career and a chilly reception from other analysts." Moreover, with respect to psychoanalytic training institutes, she adds that prior to the early 1990s, "homosexual applicants were summarily turned away; many, aware of the prevailing view, did not even bother to apply" (Goode, 1998). On the client side, LGBTQ individuals continue to report experiencing "considerable discrimination and hostility during the therapeutic process" (Bowers, Plummer, & Minichiello, 2005), as well as more insidious microaggressions (Shelton & Delgado-Romero, 2011). As psychotherapists Sherry S. McHenry and Jackie W. Johnson observe, the interaction of a therapist's homophobia and a client's internalized homophobia can yield "unconscious collusions… in self-hate" (McHenry & Johnson, 1993, p. 143).

And although he does not use this label, Crowley's intervention of choice is tantamount to conversion therapy, a practice animated by "the notion that any nonheterosexual sexual orientation is a pathology in need of a 'cure'" (Streed, Anderson, Babits, & Ferguson, 2019, p. 500). While it may come as a surprise to some, conversion therapy is hardly a thing of the past. In the United States, as of August 2019, a total of 18 states plus Puerto Rico and Washington, D.C. prohibit conversion therapy for minors—the practice remains legal in the remaining states for minors and across all states for adults on a voluntary basis (Streed, Anderson, Babits, & Ferguson, 2019).

Additionally, there remains well-documented LGBTQ bias throughout the American criminal legal system. A recent volume on the subject offers this eloquent, disquieting summary of pervasive animus and cruelty:

> The specter of criminality moves ceaselessly through the lives of LGBT people in the United States. It is the enduring product of persistent melding of homosexuality and gender nonconformity with concepts of *danger, degeneracy, disorder, deception, disease, contagion, sexual predation, depravity, subversion, encroachment, treachery, and violence...* In the realm of criminal archetypes, anxiety, fear, and dread prevail - potent emotions that can easily overpower reason.
>
> (Mogul, Ritchie, & Whitlock, 2011, p. 23)

Perhaps less expected, however, the criminal case processing and sentencing scheme that Crowley documents in 1938 also bears an uncanny resemblance to contemporary practice in courts that offer therapeutic intervention as an alternative to incarceration. As is common today, Crowley describes a relatively informal legal process, "the informal trial," in which mental health professionals offer diagnostic and treatment recommendations not as "witnesses" (e.g., not subject to cross-examination) but rather as "friends of the court" (Crowley, 1938, p. 266). Also consistent with current operations, the court is deferential to the point of view of the mental health experts and crafts a disposition that mandates treatment "instead of punishment" (p. 268). The court tacitly agrees with the clinician's assessment that there is both a sickness and a cure when it uses its power to compel treatment.

To be clear, a lack of formal legal process (e.g., due process rights to a trial, to confront witnesses, etc.) is hardly unique to specialized treatment courts. In 2017, 97.2 percent of criminal cases in the United States were resolved through plea bargains (Jones et al., 2018, p. 14). Moreover, new research estimates that only *one* out of every ten thousand misdemeanor judgements in a given year is ever "disturbed" on appeal. As the authors note, "it is no wonder that judges, prosecutors, and defense counsel can be confident that their conduct in trial court proceedings in misdemeanor cases will not be reviewed" (King & Heise, 2019, p. 1980). Ultimately, "[t]he system of mass incarceration depends almost entirely on the cooperation of those it seeks to control," observes author and law professor Michelle Alexander (Alexander, 2012). "If everyone charged with crimes suddenly exercised his constitutional rights, there would not be enough judges, lawyers or prison cells to deal with the ensuing tsunami of litigation" (Alexander, 2012).

Regardless, defense-minded critics of treatment courts have long bemoaned precisely what Crowley lauds as "the meeting of law and medicine in a common undertaking" (Crowley, 1938, p. 266). As zealous advocates, the argument goes, defense attorneys are tasked with representing their clients' wishes, even *or especially* if these wishes may not align with best interests from a clinical or treatment perspective (Meekins, 2007).

Coupled with this informality is an underlying, nonreflexive justification that any alternative to incarceration must be better for the individual than the direct and collateral harms of confinement. Crowley concludes his article on this very point:

> Sending Z to the penitentiary would have made his problem not better, but worse. With his salary stopped, how would his family have been supported? On release, he would have had to contend not only with the stigma of having been in prison, but also with the stigma of perversion... Once in the penitentiary, the other prisoners would soon have learned why he was there. During his whole stay they would have ridiculed him and called him obscene names... With knowledge of his offense, others would have desired him sexually. Z was a man of culture and refinement and such experiences could hardly fail to have had a permanently crippling effect... Due, however, to the intelligent cooperation of court and psychiatrist, Z was able to receive therapeutic treatment instead of punishment and resume his place in society.
>
> (Crowley, 1938, p. 268)

A 2016 survey of crime victims' views on incarceration echoes similar themes: "By a margin of nearly 3 to 1," the survey finds that "victims believe that prison makes people more likely to commit crimes than to rehabilitate them... and prefer holding people accountable through options beyond prison, such as rehabilitation, mental health treatment, drug treatment, community supervision, or community service" (Alliance for Safety and Justice, n.d.). But a recent report on the landscape of court-mandated community service in the United States makes clear that not all community-based options are sufficiently or consistently equitable and rehabilitative (Picard, Tallon, Lowry, & Kralstein, 2019). The same can be said for court-mandated treatment (Szalavitz, 2015).

In a similar vein, some have criticized treatment courts for being more coercive than traditional courts, especially when access to social services is conditional upon a guilty plea (Thompson, 2002, p. 37). And while legal due process and therapeutic alternatives to incarceration are neither mutually exclusive in theory nor in practice (Adler & Taylor, 2012), accounts like Crowley's raise the specter of mandated treatment as an undue constraint on individual liberty interests—albeit, in lieu of physical confinement.

The point here is certainly not to challenge the fundamental idea that incarceration is harmful and to be avoided wherever possible. We wholeheartedly agree with John Jay College of Criminal Justice professor Deborah Koetzle: "Prison is not the answer...Prison can make people worse" (Koetzle, 2018). Rather, the idea here is that there is a frequently unchecked logic of ends (avoiding incarceration) justifying the means (in Crowley's case, conversion therapy). In other words, treatment as an alternative to incarceration should be justifiable both as an improvement on something else *and* as an appropriate, normatively defensible intervention in and of itself.

This leads to a third feature of Crowley's article that resembles many current clinical practices—both inside and outside of courthouses, for that matter: hubris. Crowley is unequivocally confident that he has identified "the real underlying cause" of Mr. Z's sex acts with men (Crowley, 1938, p. 266). In his pathologizing account of Mr. Z's familial conflicts and anxieties, there is not even a mention of the possibility that Mr. Z might be a gay man stuck in an unhappy marriage to a woman in a society that criminalizes his sexuality. Nor that there may exist a constellation of factors causing Mr. Z difficulties rather than "*an* [emphasis added] underlying factor" (p. 266). And, at the risk of stating the obvious, at no point does Crowley question his own homophobic bias.

A recent American Psychological Association article on alternatives to incarceration is similarly hubristic in its framing, making the case that "[d]rug and mental health courts give certain offenders what they *really* [emphasis added] need: treatment" (Bailey, 2003). While it may very well be the case that many participants in these courts do benefit from formal treatment, it may not be the case that treatment is able to address a or *the* driving cause of their criminal justice involvement. There is a growing trend in criminal justice of recognizing a broader range of "criminogenic" factors that can drive recidivism (e.g., peers, lack of employment, familial conflict) (Bonta & Andrews, 2016). There is also an increasing awareness in criminal justice that "[t]he majority of individuals who interface with the criminal justice system - including prisons, jails and detention centers - have been exposed to traumatic events across the life-course" (Kubiak, Covington, & Hillier).

Critically, though, in addition to the importance of multidimensional clinical formulations, any diagnostic practice in the criminal justice context must account for the role of the system itself. For example, "a growing body of scholarship... views recidivism as an ecological phenomenon," notes criminal justice researcher Sarah Picard, which is "co-produced by individual and environmental risk factors" (Picard, 2019, p. 88). Picard's research finds that "living in a highly policed area could act as a gateway back into the criminal justice system for individuals otherwise at low risk for a new arrest" (Picard, 2019, p. 62). Writing in the University of Pennsylvania Law Review, Colorado Judge Morris B. Hoffman doubles-down on non-clinical explanations for justice system involvement: "In Denver, where I preside, drug filings almost tripled one year after the institution of our drug court compared with one year before. A big part of the net-widening phenomenon is pretty straightforward: police and prosecutors are no longer trying to detect crime; they are trolling for patients" (Hoffman, 2011, p. 131). Just as Crowley elides oppressive systemic variables in his analysis of Mr. Z, there is a similar tendency in contemporary practice to reduce justice involvement to "poor individual choices or deficiencies" (Kramer, Rajah, & Sung, 2013, p. 553).

Beyond Crowley

What is to be done? Accepting the abolitionist critique that the criminal legal system is inherently harmful as constructed, how might clinicians still practice in a manner aimed at appreciably reducing harm? To this end, what lessons can we learn from Crowley to inform the present moment?

One deceptively simple takeaway from Crowley is to practice hypervigilance with respect to potential clinician bias. The problem, of course, is that there is often an interpenetration of bias and a clinical viewpoint or theoretical mooring. In Crowley's case, it is unclear where his homophobic bias ends and his clinical perspective begins (and there is no indication of whether he is interested in Mr. Z's self-determination). As discussed above, even Crowley's diagnostic approach imports a policy position on the criminalization of homosexuality. This latter point is critical: Crowley's expert clinical perspective, to which the judge is largely deferential, *is* also a legal position. While Crowley's case is problematic, it also illustrates the power that clinicians wield in courtrooms. This power is a potential force for good (e.g., the understanding of how trauma and oppression affect behavior and finding ways to bring this insight to bear on courtroom proceedings).

While by no means a panacea, some literature has noted the importance of recognizing systemic biases in social service provision and the potential effects of this recognition on criminal law. In the context of racial bias, for example, George Washington University law professor Cynthia Lee argues that "[t]he problem is that ignoring racial difference can actually exacerbate the effects of implicit racial bias. It is when we are not paying attention to race that we are most vulnerable to racial stereotyping" (Lee, 2014, p. 94). As key actors with an increasingly large presence in the criminal legal system, social workers, clinicians, and other mental health professionals may alter the discourse around systemic biases by recognizing them openly in their work.

Another takeaway from Crowley is the critical interplay between bias and the clinical hubris that serves to entrench and perpetuate it in practice. Perhaps a helpfully humbling reference point for clinicians is the meta-analytic research on psychotherapy outcomes that finds cross-cutting relational factors (e.g., empathy, alliance, positive regard) dwarf any specific techniques, strategies, theories, or models (Wampold, 2015). Arguably, disinvestment from—or less rigidity about—clinical theories and treatment models (and dogmas) could create more room for critical self-reflection and the identification of biases.

And while the eradication of bias is a Herculean lift unto itself [and, as it were, the source of some debate around the efficacy of implicit bias tests (Weir, 2016)], there is also the challenge of broadening the clinical frame to recognize the harms wrought by the system(s) itself. Such an ecological approach "offers a novel framework for addressing the high rates and broad range of criminogenic and clinical needs among [individuals] in the context of their lived experience rather than divorced from it (a potential pitfall of some cognitive behavioral therapy practice)" (White et al., 2018, p. iv).

As a threshold matter, clinicians must be willing to challenge social injustice rather than—*a la* Crowley—reinforce it by pathologizing the behavior of individuals. Crowley utterly fails to challenge the oppression of gay men. Instead, he validates the homophobia embedded within the law by purporting to be capable of making Mr. Z accommodate the homophobic norm. Notably, this calls to mind Judith Herman's seminal critique of Freud's failure to acknowledge his female patients' reports of childhood sexual abuse. Herman recounts the genesis of psychoanalysis as the willful denial of a widespread social injustice:

> Hysteria was so common among women that if his patients' stories were true, and if his theory was correct, he would be forced to conclude that what he called 'perverted acts against children' were endemic, not only among the proletariat of Paris... but also among the respectable bourgeois families of Vienna... This idea was simply unacceptable... Faced with this dilemma, Freud stopped listening to his female patients... Out of the ruins of the traumatic theory of hysteria, Freud created psychoanalysis. The dominant psychological theory of the next century was founded in the denial of women's reality.
>
> (Herman, 1992, p. 14)

As Herman contends, Freud chose to pathologize his patients—"as if the exploitative situation were a fulfillment of [Dora's] desire" (p. 14)—rather than confront the social, systemic etiology of their anxieties. Crowley did the same.

To aid a potential paradigm shift, to orient clinicians in the criminal legal system toward the harms of the system itself, one potentially useful source is the work of disability advocates to replace the medical model with a social one. Whereas the former "conceptualized disability as a tragedy or problem localized in an individual body or mind," the latter posited disability "as a social phenomenon caused by social oppression and prejudices" (Beaudry, 2016, p. 210). Echoing a through line of this chapter, notes from a 1975 meeting of The Union of the Physically Impaired Against Segregation and The Disability Alliance call out the harms of overly-individualized explanations for people affected and ensnared by systems:

> For us as disabled people it is absolutely vital that we get this question of the cause of disability quite straight, because on the answer depends the crucial matter of where we direct our main energies in the struggle for change. We shall clearly get nowhere if our efforts are chiefly directed not at the cause of our oppression, but instead at one of the symptoms.
>
> (Union of the Physically Impaired Against Segregation and the Disability Alliance, 1975)

To be clear, this is not to suggest categorically that individuals mandated to treatment through the criminal legal system do not present with a spectrum of cognizable clinical needs. It is, however, to argue that the way we understand and attempt to respond to these needs must account for the role(s) played and harms wrought by the system itself—as well as how the discursive context, the ecology, may *always already* bias our assessments and clinical actions (Althusser, 2014).

Court and Couch Revisited

Ultimately, this chapter can be read as a rejoinder to Michel Foucault's trivialization of "that safest and most discrete of spaces, between the couch and discourse" (Foucault, 1976, p. 5). For better and for worse, clinicians, in fact, have tremendous influence on the broader social discourse—including its normative boundaries and their attendant legal mechanisms. In the context of criminal justice reform, clinicians will continue to wield influence, both through their direct practices and their more interstitial engagements with stakeholders. Admittedly, it feels unsatisfying to conclude here without a new model or protocol or some set of strategies for the effective importation of social justice into the therapeutic process. Instead, what we have from Crowley is a sobering (and urgent) reminder that the psychoanalytic or clinical sensibility, left unchecked, has the potential to perpetuate and even further entrench the most harmful aspects of the social order. It bears repeating that the editor of *Psychiatry*, Harry Stack Sullivan, a gay man (though this was not widely known by his contemporaries), together and with the William Alanson White Foundation, held up Crowley's article in a journal intended to capture the leading-edge of interdisciplinary practice—with all the contradictions that involved. Unwitting as this may have been, Crowley's project cannot be rationalized (then or now) along the lines of sublimation; this is about the indefensible exercise of oppression and the need for clinicians to confront it.

Note

1. We would like to thank Joy Ming King (Wesleyan University) and Raquel Delerme (Center for Court Innovation) for invaluable research support. Deep appreciation to Sophia English, Yolaine Menyard, and Anna Pomper for their thoughtful comments on an earlier draft.

References

Adler, J. & Taylor, B. (2012). Minding the elephant: Criminal defense practice in community courts. *The Judge's Journal*, 51, 10–15. Retrieved from https://www.courtinnovation.org/sites/default/files/documents/JJ_SP12_AdlerTaylor-1.pdf

Alexander, M. (2012, March 10). Go to trial: Crash the justice system. *The New York Times*. Retrieved from https://www.nytimes.com/2012/03/11/opinion/sunday/go-to-trial-crash-the-justice-system.html

Allen, F. A. (1978). The decline of the rehabilitative ideal in American criminal justice. *Cleveland State Law Review*, 27, 147–156. Retrieved from https://engagedscholarship.csuohio.edu/clevstlrev/vol27/iss2/3/

Allen, L. (1955, March–April). Reformers can be cruel. *Mattachine Review*, 2, 31. Retrieved from http://digitalassets.lib.berkeley.edu/sfbagals/Mattachine_Review/1955_Mattachine_Mar-Apr.pdf

Alliance for Safety and Justice (n.d.). *Crime survivors speak: The first-ever nation survey of victim's views on safety and justice*. Retrieved from http://www.allianceforsafetyandjustice.org/wp-content/uploads/documents/Crime%20Survivors%20Speak%20Report.pdf

Althusser, L. (2014). *On the Reproduction of Capitalism: Ideology and Ideological State Apparatuses*. Brooklyn, New York: Verso.

American Psychoanalytic Association (2019, June 21). *American Psychoanalytic Association issues overdue apology to LGBTQ Community* [press release]. Retrieved from http://www.apsa.org/content/news-apsaa-issues-overdue-apology-lgbtq-community

American University & Bureau of Justice Assistance (2008). *Challenges and solutions to implementing problem-solving courts from the traditional court management perspective.* Retrieved from https://www.bja.gov/Publications/AU_ProbSolvCourts.pdf

Bailey, D. S. (2003, July/August). Alternatives to incarceration: Drug and mental health courts give certain offenders what they really need: treatment. *Monitor on Psychology*, 34(7). Retrieved from https://www.apa.org/monitor/julaug03/alternatives

Beaudry, J. S. (2016). Beyond (models of) disability?. *Journal of Medical Philosophy*, 41(2), 210–228. doi:10.1093/jmp/jhv063

Bowers, R., Plummer, D., & Minichiello, V. (2005). Homophobia in counselling practice. *International Journal for the Advancement of Counselling*, 27(3), 471–489. doi: 10.1007/s10447-005-8207-7

Cavendish, M. (2010). *Sex and Society* (p. 825). Singapore: Marshall Cavendish Corporation.

Crowley, R. M. (1935). The courts and psychiatry. *Psychiatry: Journal of the Biology and the Pathology of Interpersonal Relations*, 1, 265–268.

Dailey, A. C. (2017). *Law and the Unconscious: A Psychoanalytic Perspective.* New Haven: Yale University Press.

D'Emilio, J. (1983). *Sexual Politics, Sexual Communities: The Making of a Homosexual Minority in the United States, 1940–1970.* Chicago: University of Chicago Press.

Eskridge Jr., W. N. (1997). Law and the construction of the closet: American regulation of same-sex intimacy, 1880–1946. *Iowa Law Review*, 82(4), 1007–1136.

Foucault, M. (1976). *The History of Sexuality, Volume 1: An Introduction.* New York, NY: Random House.

Foucault, M. (1977). *Discipline and Punish: The Birth of the Prison.* New York, NY: Pantheon Books.

Gilmore, R. W. & Kilgore, J. (2019, June). The case for abolition. The Marshall Project. Retrieved from https://www.themarshallproject.org/2019/06/19/the-case-for-abolition

Goode, E. (1998, December 12). On gay issue, psychoanalysis treats itself. *The New York Times.* Retrieved from https://www.nytimes.com/1998/12/12/arts/on-gay-issue-psychoanalysis-treats-itself.html

Herman, J. (1992). *Trauma and Recovery.* New York, NY: Basic Books.

Hoffman, M. B. (2001). The rehabilitative ideal and the drug court reality. *Federal Sentencing Reporter*, 14(3–4), 172–178. doi: 10.1525/fsr.2001.14.3-4.172

Hoffman, M. B. (2011). Problem-solving courts and the psychological error. *University of Pennsylvania Law Review PENNumbra*, 160, 131. Retrieved from https://www.pennlawreview.com/online/160-U-Pa-L-Rev-PENNumbra-129.pdf

Jones, R. et al. (2018). *The Trial Penalty: The Sixth Amendment Right to Trial on the Verge of Extinction and How to Save It.* Retrieved from National Association of Criminal Defense Lawyers website: https://www.nacdl.org/Document/TrialPenaltySixthAmendmentRighttoTrialNearExtinct

King, N. J. & Heise, M. (2019). Misdemeanor appeals. *Boston University Law Review*, 99, 1933–1993.

Koetzle, D. (2018). *Addressing crime and drug use through community bases interventions.* TedxOneonta. Available from https://www.ted.com/talks/deborah_koetzle_koetzle_addressing_crime_and_drug_use_through_community_based_interventions

Kramer, R., Rajah, V., & Sung, H. E. (2013). Neoliberal prisons and cognitive treatment: Calibrating the subjectivity of incarcerated young men to economic inequalities. *Theoretical Criminology*, 17(4). doi: 10.1177/1362480613497780

Kubiak, S. P., Covington, S. S., & Hillier, C. *Trauma-informed corrections.* https://www.centerforgenderandjustice.org/assets/files/soical-work-chapter-7-trauma-informed-corrections-final.pdf

Lanzer, I. A. (1948, May–June). Forensic social case work: An analytical survey. *Journal of Criminal Law and Criminology (1931–1951)*, 39(1), 34–48.

Lee, C. (2014). (E)Racing Trayvon Martin. *Ohio State Journal of Criminal Law*, 12(1), 91–113. Retrieved from https://kb.osu.edu/bitstream/handle/1811/73474/OSJCL_V12N1_091.pdf?sequence=1&isAllowed=y

Manuscripts and Archives Division, The New York Public Library. (1964). *Penalties for Sex Offenses in the United States.* Retrieved from http://digitalcollections.nypl.org/items/671159d8-0456-a33c-e040-e00a180655cb

Marlowe, D. B., Hardin, C. D., & Fox, C. L. (2016). *Painting the Current Picture: A national report on drug courts and other problem-solving courts in the United States.* Retrieved from National Drug Court Institute website: https://www.ndci.org/wp-content/uploads/2016/05/Painting-the-Current-Picture-2016.pdf

McHenry, S. & Johnson, J. (1993). Homophobia in the therapist and gay or lesbian client: Conscious and unconscious collusion in self-hate. *Psychotherapy: Theory, Research, Practice, Training*, 30(1), 141–151. doi:10.1037/0033-3204.30.1.141

Meekins, T. A. (2007). Risky business: Criminal specialty courts and the ethical obligations of the zealous criminal defender. *Berkeley Journal of Criminal Law*, 12, 75–126.

Mogul, J. L., Ritchie, A. J., & Whitlock, K. (2011). *Queer (In)justice: The Criminalization of LGBT People in the United States.* Boston, MA: Beacon Press.

Pearl, B. (2018, June 27). *Ending the war on drugs: By the numbers.* Retrieved from Center for American Progress website: https://www.americanprogress.org/issues/criminal-justice/reports/2018/06/27/452819/ending-war-drugs-numbers/

Picard, S. (2019). *Neighborhood ecology and recidivism: A case study in NYC* (unpublished doctoral dissertation). New York: The City University of New York.

Picard. S., Tallon, J. A., Lowry, M., & Kralstein, D. (2019). *Court ordered community service: A national perspective.* Retrieved from Center for Court Innovation website: https://www.courtinnovation.org/sites/default/files/media/document/2019/community_service_report_11052019_0.pdf

Pierceson, J. et al., eds. (2010). *Same-Sex Marriage in the Americas: Policy Innovation for Same-Sex Relationships.* Maryland: Lexington Books.

Shelton, K. & Delgado-Romero, E. A. (2011). Sexual orientation microaggressions: The experience of lesbian, gay, bisexual, and queer clients in psychotherapy. *Journal of Counseling Psychology, 58*(2), 210–221. doi: 10.1037/a0022251

Streed, C. G., Anderson, S., Babits, C., & Ferguson, M. (2019). Changing medical practice, not patients – putting an end to conversion therapy. *New England Journal of Medicine, 381*(6), 500–502. doi: 10.1056/NEJMp1903161

Szalavitz, M. (2015, May 18). How America overdosed on drug courts. *Pacific Standard Magazine.* Retrieved from https://psmag.com/news/how-america-overdosed-on-drug-courts

Thompson, A. C. (2002). Courting disorder: Some thoughts on community courts. *Washington University Journal of Law and Policy,* 10, 63–103.

Thompson, D. & Beam, A. (2019, July). National Leaders start group for bipartisan criminal justice reform. *Christian Science Monitor.* Retrieved from https://www.csmonitor.com/USA/Justice/2019/0723/National-leaders-start-group-for-bipartisan-criminal-justice-reform

Union of the Physically Impaired Against Segregation and the Disability Alliance (1975). *Fundamental Principals of Disability (summary of discussion held on 22nd November, 1975).* Retrieved from https://disability-studies.leeds.ac.uk/wp-content/uploads/sites/40/library/UPIAS-fundamental-principles.pdf

Vitiello, M. (2013). Alternatives to incarceration: Why is California lagging behind? *Georgia State University Law Review, 28*(4), 1273–1312. Retrieved from https://readingroom.law.gsu.edu/gsulr/vol28/iss4/10?utm_source=readingroom.law.gsu.edu%2Fgsulr%2Fvol28%2Fiss4%2F10&utm_medium=PDF&utm_campaign=PDFCoverPages

Waggoner, W. H. (1984, November 1). Dr. Ralph Manning Crowley, Psychoanalyst, is dead at 78. *The New York Times.* Retrieved from https://www.nytimes.com/1984/11/01/obituaries/dr-ralph-manning-crowley-psychoanalyst-is-dead-at-78.html

Wampold, B. E. (2015). How important are the common factors in psychotherapy? An update. *World Psychiatry,* 14(3), 270–277. doi: 10.1002/wps.20238

Weir, K. (2016, December). Adoption of implicit bias tests is 'hasty'. *Monitor on Psychology,* 47(11). Retrieved from http://www.apa.org/monitor/2016/12/policing-sidebar

White, E., et al. (2018). *Toward an evidence-based response to misdemeanors.* Retrieved from Center for Court Innovation website: https://www.courtinnovation.org/sites/default/files/media/document/2018/upout_misdemeanors.pdf

Chapter 7

Immigrants in Our Own Country
Responsibility Towards the Past and Future of Interpersonal Psychoanalysis

Orsolya Hunyady

"The anthropological research may be somewhat obscure – never heard of it - and the reference to 'Totem and Taboo' is strikingly missing." Paraphrased, this was Sigmund Freud's take on Edith Weigert-Vowinckel's paper entitled "The Cult and Mythology of the Magna Mater from the Standpoint of Psychoanalysis" (Weigert-Vowinkel, 1938). Freud's response temporarily shattered the young German psychoanalyst's heartfelt hopes for publication and acknowledgment (see Holmes, 2010, p. 13). Weigert's former analyst and mentor, Carl Muller-Braunschweig, had suggested that she contact Freud, praising the paper, which indeed is extensive, deeply researched, and a clear contribution to the field. Weigert (1894–1982) interrogates and expands on the Western cultural context in which Freud and psychoanalysis talk about Oedipal dynamics and the relations between the sexes.

Weigert's correspondence with Freud about the paper took place in 1937, by which time the National Socialist regime in Germany was already well established. Following their assumption of power in 1933, Hitler and the Nazi party quickly made psychoanalysis a target. Weigert, a psychiatrist, trained at the famed Berlin Psychoanalytic Institute. In 1935, Weigert and her husband, who was of Jewish descent, left Germany for Turkey and later found their way to the United States. Freud himself would soon be forced to do the same, fleeing for England after the Anschluss in March 1938 that 'united' Austria with Germany. At the time, the European and international psychoanalytic scene had solidified into a network of societies,

DOI: 10.4324/9781003270355-8

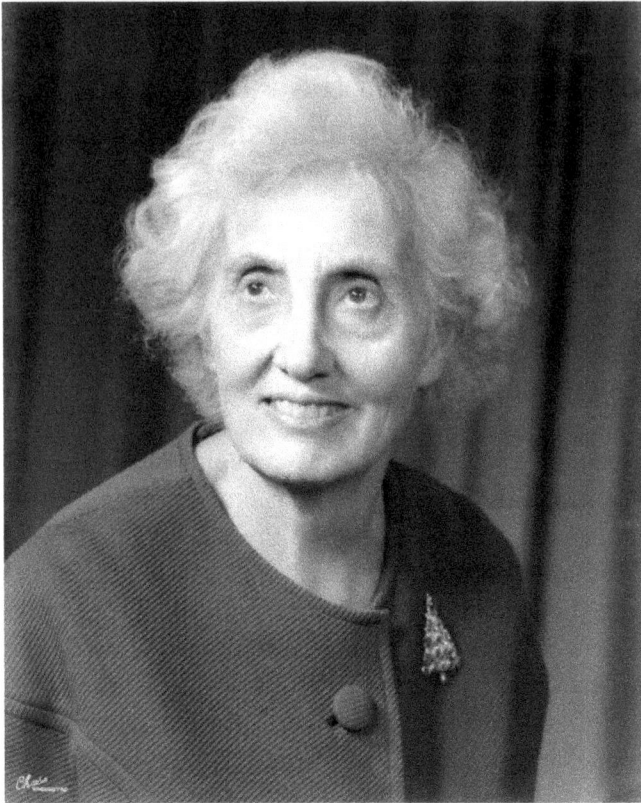

Figure 7 Edith Weigert, 1946, © Washington Baltimore Center for Psychoanalysis.

institutes, and associated journals, and Freud's negative judgment of Weigert's paper could have presented an insurmountable obstacle in getting it published at all.

In her paper, Weigert delved deeply into the mythology of Asia Minor, examining its matriarchal societies – and mother-son relations, in particular – to see what happened with feelings of guilt, competitiveness, fear, and aggression under these conditions. She observed a parallel to penis envy in men: an envy of women's reproductive capabilities, and highlighted the prevalence of self-castration as a religious ritual, a means to eliminate adulthood and become (by a self-sacrificing act) a child in psychic fusion with the Great Mother for eternity (see also Osman, 2004). Weigert underlines that sin in these cultures had to do with separation and independence having a separate identity. She further argues that circumcision is a tamed, transformed version of the original self-castration. Sacrificing one's self or a part of one's self to one's God remained a prevalent theme in the Bible, she continues, that otherwise can be considered an important milestone in the process of suppression of female deities in religious texts and rituals. Even though a transition to patriarchy was completed, the mother theme did not stop to pervade religious thought and practices (Weigert-Vowinkel, 1938). In other words, Weigert sought to point out that the conceptual Mother is (or remains) as foundational in the psyche as the conceptual Father, as it had been encapsulated in the notion of the Oedipal complex. She thus suggested the subversion of Freudian dogma through an interdisciplinary, anthropological approach.

Despite his negative judgment, Freud did not actively interfere with the publication of the manuscript, which was eventually accepted by *Imago* – but ultimately failed to be published because of its 'political implications' (Holmes, 2010, p. 14). Muller-Braunschweig, who at this point seemed to have become an explicit advocate for Weigert, raised the issue with Freud six months after Weigert's exchange with him. He described to Freud how upset she was as a result of Freud's disapproval, and asked for more sympathy and a reason for his rejecting attitude. Muller-Braunschweig himself was quite interested in ideas at the intersection of psychoanalysis and anthropology, a topic on which he had published during the 1920s and early 1930s. In contrast to Weigert and Freud, Muller-Braunschweig was not threatened by Nazi rule. On the contrary, following 1933, he willingly took charge of the German Psychoanalytic Society with the explicit mission of adapting it to the regime's National Socialist ideology.

Since Weigert culturally contextualized the Oedipal Complex, stripping it from its universal status, and since she refused as well to reduce religion to its neurotic roots and defensive functions, it is not very surprising that her work provoked Freud's dismay. As we know, Freud never took well to challenges that questioned the main tenets of psychoanalysis, despite his own remarkable ability to evolve his thinking and theories in light of new observations. In answer to Muller-Braunschweig's question, Freud said that in his opinion, it would have been satisfactory for Weigert to explain Magna Mater and self-castration simply as part of the Oedipal Complex; he believed "that a woman's dominance must have something to do with the removal of the father, and self-castration with repentance" – essentially dismissing Weigert's points altogether (Holmes, 2010, p. 14). Weigert, however, would not be dissuaded. She continued to work on publishing the manuscript, which was translated into English and finally reached publication in 1938, appearing in the first volume of the radical new journal *Psychiatry: Journal of the Biology and the Pathology of Interpersonal Relations*.

For Weigert, getting her paper published in English was an intentional act of preparation for her immigration to the United States. Leaving Germany was a decision necessitated by her husband's persecution by the Nazis, which first took the couple to Turkey, before finding a permanent home in Washington. Kemal Ataturk had requested Weigert's husband's assistance with creating a modern statute of employment law in Turkey, and Weigert joined him with their two-year-old son, hoping that 'things will blow over soon enough' in Germany for them to be able to return (Holmes, 2010, p. 12). Weigert had an incredibly active few years in Ankara, finding company among many other ex-pats, becoming instrumental in introducing psychoanalysis in Turkey and becoming a prolific writer, notably writing the Magna Mater article during this period. Nazism certainly did not 'blow over' by the time her husband completed his assignment, and thus the Weigert family made another move to the United States. Reportedly, these moves were hard on Weigert, and despite her success and deep professional and personal involvement in the psychoanalytic scene, and despite the successful preservation of her connections in Europe [unlike her Jewish colleagues, she never resigned from the German Psychoanalytical Society (DPG)], she went through several quite severe depressive episodes as a consequence of her forced emigration (Holmes, 2010, p. 16). Her emotional hardships, I believe, speak to the inherent strains that an immigration poses on a person, especially if it is brought on by persecution and political instability. Weigert's circumstances, reception, way of entry into a new culture, and professional scene were as smooth, well-prepared, and strongly invited as possible, and yet she still suffered quite intensely as a result of the change.

Weigert's affinities, sensibilities, and personal history led her to appreciate and focus on the role of actual historical developments, societal and social structures in the genesis and operation of the human psyche. Once she had been forced out of the comfort of her native country, led by her intellectual interests, she turned her attention to interdisciplinary studies using anthropological data, eventually leading her to question psychoanalytic dogma. Weigert's immigration put her in direct touch with several other cultures, all of which informed her psychoanalytic theorizing and practice, extending traditional psychoanalytic thought beyond its old boundaries. In what follows, we will examine up close her own journey towards becoming an accepted psychoanalyst in the United States. We will pay special attention to the historical context and the role Weigert and other European émigré psychoanalysts played in the development of the interpersonal school.

Weigert, Sullivan, and the Interpersonal School of Psychiatry

In 1938, Weigert's first stop in the United States was New York City with the ultimate goal of moving to Washington, DC in order to accommodate her husband's career constraints. Weigert was referred to Harry Stack Sullivan by Karen Horney whom Weigert knew from their Berlin days, and once in Washington, she rekindled her acquaintance with Frieda Fromm-Reichmann with whom she developed a close friendship soon after that. The publication of her Magna Mater paper in the same year was quickly followed by other professional successes, such as becoming a teaching analyst and member of the Washington educational committee in 1939 (Holmes, 2010, p. 14), where she continued to exert influence.

Harry Stack Sullivan was one of the most influential and controversial figures in the Washington psychoanalytic scene at the time of Weigert's immigration. He actively participated in the foundation of the William Alanson White Psychoanalytic (after 1937, Psychiatric) Foundation in 1933, and later of the Washington School of Psychiatry in 1936. In 1938, he helped found and served as the first editor of the journal *Psychiatry*. After the end of the World War II, he helped establish the World Federation for Mental Health. Sullivan, like many in his circle, came to psychoanalysis through studying and treating psychoses–an endeavor that his more classical-conventional colleagues in Europe would not undertake. As we know, he eventually developed a systematic theory of development that underlined the interpersonal determinants of personality and emphasized the cultural elements in mental disorders. He uniquely combined psychoanalytic insights with observations from the social sciences, inspired by such thinkers as Edward Sapir, a cultural anthropologist; Harold Lasswell, a political scientist; and George Herbert Mead, Robert Ezra Park, and W. I. Thomas, internationally distinguished sociologists. This interdisciplinary approach to the matters of human psychological functioning was reflected in the very structure of the William Alanson White Foundation, which originally had three departments: biology, social sciences, and psychiatry. It was also reflected in the mission of the journal *Psychiatry*, where it was made explicit that papers were to be accepted from the biological and social sciences as much as from psychiatry, and that these papers address an audience that includes "all serious students of human living" (William Alanson White Psychiatric Foundation, 1938, p. ii). This interdisciplinary attitude went beyond emphasizing an individual's inextricable embeddedness in his various contexts; it pointed to the emergence of the individual out of the intersection of these contexts.

The breaching of conventional boundaries that characterized the early interpersonal school both in terms of diagnostic categories being treated, and of diverse theoretical sources applied to psychoanalytic thought, struck Sullivan's more classically oriented colleagues as an attempt to 'dilute' psychoanalysis through eclecticism, and by the mid-1940s, great personal and intellectual animosity developed, creating deep fault-lines within the Washington-Baltimore community. With Lucile Dooley and Ernest Hadley on one side, and Sullivan, Freida Fromm-Reichmann, and Dexter Bullard on the other, the battle for psychoanalysis' (maybe) soul, and for its social standing (certainly) began. The former group, leaning towards ego-psychology, wanted to set up the training institute as 'purely Freudian,' whereas the latter group considered the modifications to conventional theory and practice to be essential and necessary adaptations to changing times (Bryce, 2020).

The intellectual debate between the two camps was magnified by interpersonal animosities, and by different visions of the future of psychoanalysis as a discipline. The first group argued for more exclusivity and preservation of 'standards' and 'boundaries,' while the second group argued for inclusiveness and flexibility, even at the potential cost of being considered less rigorous. The power struggle culminated when Jenny Waelder-Hall, who had previously worked closely with Anna Freud, joined the organization in 1943. Donald Burnham (1978) suggested that "it is tempting to view Waelder-Hall and Sullivan not only as eloquent spokesmen but as literal personifications of Vienna orthodoxy and American eclecticism and of the difficulty, if not impossibility, of reconciling the two" (p. 102). Inevitably – and fitting right into a long line of defections, splits, and schisms (Eisold, 1994) – the institute officially broke into two in 1947, and the APA eventually recognized a separate Baltimore Psychoanalytic Society with its own educational program. It took two more years for the two institutes to fully separate and establish themselves individually.

Amidst all this turmoil, Weigert took Sullivan's side for various reasons, I imagine. For one, she strongly believed in the possibility and meaningfulness of treating schizophrenic patients with psychotherapy, which naturally aligned her with the more innovative, interpersonal group. She also had her differences with classical Freudian theory, as we saw apropos of the Magna Mater article, and all this contributed to her strong personal connections to Horney, Fromm-Reichmann, and Sullivan himself. This – coupled with an aversion to oppressive attitudes of those in power – probably determined her response to the situation. Weigert, however, was trained classically and never disavowed her intellectual roots. Unlike her above-mentioned colleagues, her tendency was to work consistently against division, and she often took on the role of 'translating' between the Freudian and interpersonal schools, highlighting the ways in which their notions are compatible, even similar (Holmes, 2010). Weigert was respected, by and large, by both sides, and never became the focus of harsh criticism nor severe conflict. In this way, we might say that Weigert was not your typical prominent psychoanalyst, and yet she was successful and was actively as well as publicly involved in all aspects of the psychoanalytic scene.

While the Washington circle was facing up to its irreconcilable differences, similar dynamics surfaced in the New York psychoanalytic world. Karen Horney and Clara Thompson – representing the interpersonal-cultural trend within the New York Psychoanalytic Institute – developed personal and professional antagonisms with Lawrence Kubie among others. Continuing the general trend of splits and fragmentation, in 1941, Horney and Thompson, along with H. Ephron, B. Robbins, and S. Kelman, left the Institute and founded the Association for the Advancement of Psychoanalysis, and its journal, the *American Journal of Psychoanalysis*, which quickly became popular among candidates and attracted more high-profile faculty. According to Sue Shapiro (2017), this break resulted not simply from intellectual – shall we say, ideological – differences between the classical and cultural groups, but also from envy surrounding the cultural school's popularity, and a need to appear respectable and beyond reproach, which Horney's sexual history with younger men and students/supervisees/analysands seriously undermined.

The web of complicated personal relationships, disagreement, pain, hurt, and envy, lie right under the surface, ready to burst, and plagued Horney's Institute. Yet another irreconcilable conflict developed between Horney and Erich Fromm, ultimately leading to another split two years later, out of which the William Alanson White Institute was born. Erich Fromm, Clara Thompson, Frieda Fromm-Reichmann, David Rioch and Janet Rioch, along with Sullivan, spearheaded this new organization, which originally was a satellite institution of the William Alanson White Foundation of Washington, DC. Continuing to center around Sullivan's ideas and an interpersonal sensibility, the new institute began its own struggle to fully establish its identity and be acknowledged as a legitimate psychoanalytic training and research entity.

Immigration: Its Contribution to Psychoanalytic Developments in the United States

In keeping with the central tenets of the cultural-interpersonal focus within psychoanalysis, we are obligated, I feel, to take a look at the geopolitical context in which all these events unfolded, so as to appreciate the role that individual immigrants, as well as immigration as such, played in the fate and identity of the interpersonal school, and more generally, of psychoanalysis in the United States. Let's start with the host environment. Abraham Brill started the first private practice in the United States and founded the New York Psychoanalytic Society in 1911 (Shapiro, 2017). Unlike Freud, who sought to distinguish psychoanalysis from the field of psychiatry, Brill saw a path to legitimacy and acknowledgment in linking psychoanalysis with psychiatry. According to Shapiro (referencing Richards, 2006), the main motivation for restricting the practice of psychoanalysis to those who earned a medical degree was to ensure prestige and respectability for the profession, and financial considerations played only a secondary role, though not a negligible one, of course. Brill and his contemporaries were aware that in order for psychoanalysis to take hold, they needed to create demand for it as well as a supply of home-grown analysts to meet this demand – tying psychoanalysis to medicine took care of both. The discipline was still young and fragile when the rise of Nazi Germany in Europe necessitated mass emigration. Despite their tangible apprehension and anxiety of 'being taken over,' many American and English colleagues became instrumental in helping European Jewish analysts to leave their respective countries.

The medicalization of psychoanalysis had a strong impact on the lives of these immigrants because they were unable to teach or supervise in this country unless they re-trained as doctors. This situation was particularly detrimental to women, because many medical schools would not accept them, and quotas existed for Jews, as well. The immigrants were often moved to secondary locations where few psychoanalysts had yet to establish their practices, and they were also required to become licensed in those states that they were told to settle in – sometimes a grueling process. Any European immigrant analysts could be disqualified if their original training analysis had not been done by a medical professional (Shapiro, 2017). And of course, it was not only the psychoanalytic circles that treated the arriving immigrants with ambivalence, either. In the United States, antisemitism was running high at the time; suspicion surrounded German speaking newcomers, and the FBI was keen to hunt down all real or assumed communist sympathizers.

As for the immigrants themselves, they were in reality *refugees* who had to contend with the triple trauma of having been forced to abandon their homes, of having war tear up their land, and of having to lose Freud, as well, to whom a lot of them had personal connections along with professional identifications. The United States represented physical safety and hope for a new beginning, but it fell somewhat short from the safe haven and the welcoming environment that the immigrants might have looked for. Immigration under all circumstances brings up many difficulties; having been persecuted and thus becoming a refugee carries even more extreme challenges (Parens, 2001). Loss and mourning are profound experiences associated with all forms of immigration (Akhtar, 1999). As Ainslie et al. (2013) point out, building on Antokoletz's (1994) work, these losses do not involve only the familiar physical spaces, the actual relationships, and the culturally predictable way-of-doing-things that the immigrants parted with, but also "the version of the self that was, of necessity, left behind in one's country of origin [...] Immigration not only dislocates individuals from specific environmental contexts but also disrupts the *coherence* and *continuity of self-experience*" (Ainslie et al., 2013, p. 666, emphasis added). One aspect of this lost self-experience, most relevant for psychoanalytic practice, is the strong ability to clearly articulate one's thoughts and feelings and eloquently discuss complex observations and ideas. Even this became difficult for some émigrés as they had to express themselves in an entirely new language upon arrival in the United States (Thompson, 2012).

The immigrants thus had two related tasks: taking in and attempting to adapt to a new culture and environment, as well as repairing the fractures and discontinuities (of the self), or at least attenuating to the consequences of this fragmentation. Certain émigré analysts tried to accomplish this by finding residence in familiar landscapes, recreating their old living environment in its physical manifestations as much as possible (see Thompson, 2012). Many expressed this tendency through rigidifying their psychoanalytic method in terms of teaching and technique, through becoming more restrictive in their attitudes towards 'lay analysts' who were not trained medically, and through siding with the ego-psychologists as a result of their resolve to protect and continue a dogmatic version of Freud's intellectual legacy. As Nellie L. Thompson points out:

> These émigrés belonged to a generation trained in the 1920s and 1930s during a period when Freud made his final contributions, including *Beyond the Pleasure Principle, Group Psychology and the Analysis of the Ego, The Ego and the Id, Inhibitions, Symptoms and Anxiety*, and *New Introductory Lectures*. These momentous

theoretical developments presented this generation of analysts with new avenues for investigation, and the exciting possibility that their contributions could significantly advance and consolidate psychoanalytic theory and technique.

(Thompson, 2012, p. 24)

Consequently, these émigrés saw joining up with ego-psychologists as an avenue to preserve their early hopes and aspirations and to find continuity both in terms of the direction of psychoanalysis' development and their own sense of self.

The psychoanalytic institutes became for most refugees the main source of a new identity, further increasing their investment in it and their rigidity in response to any change that was proposed to the prevailing system. Modifications to Freud's theory were unwelcome in these circles, however outdated the theory may have seemed to some. A good example of Freud's own cultural limitation in theorizing is encapsulated in his ideas about female development, of course. Freud, as we have seen in his response to Weigert's (1938) Magna Mater article, defined femininity entirely in relation to masculinity, viewing female sexuality in terms of deficiency; women in general were characterized as intellectually and morally inferior to men, while their role in child development was understated or ignored (Ponder, 2007). Many challenged these views by the 1930s and 40s, notably Karen Horney, one of the earlier feminist psychoanalytic theoreticians, and an immigrant herself. But the calcification of theory, the rigidity of identifications, coupled with heightened concerns for respectability, inevitably led to the rejection of these challenges and criticisms, ultimately making the splitting of the psychoanalytic scene and institutes inevitable.

Horney, however, was one of those immigrants who brought with her quite unconventional sensibilities. These analysts' own need to deal with their refugee status and experience, their own process of emotional adaptation, including the preservation of continuity in self, set them instead on the path of championing culturally and socially focused ideas within psychoanalysis in contrast to the focus on internal individual pathology. Dale Ortmeyer (1997) talks about two distinct groups of theorists who eventually came together to form the interpersonal school. One encompasses Sullivan, Clara Thompson, and Ferenczi – the other Erich Fromm, Frieda

Fromm-Reichmann, and Karen Horney from Berlin and Frankfurt. Sullivan first heard Clara Thompson lecture at the Phipps Clinic of Johns Hopkins University, and they became friends soon after. He also heard Ferenczi speak in New York during the late 1920s, and discussed in depth his ideas during Ferenczi's visit to Washington (Ortmeyer, 1997). To close the circle, Sullivan sent Clara to be analyzed by Ferenczi in Budapest, the mutual influence that developed among them can be easily traced in their ideas.

With respect to Erich Fromm and Freida Fromm-Reichmann, once his brief analysis was terminated with her, they got married. Both were trained at the Berlin Psychoanalytic Institute, where Horney was a founding member and on faculty, and where Weigert also trained. Fromm concluded from his observations of his study of German workers during 1929 to 1931 that their lack of well-defined character as either democratic or authoritarian rendered them highly vulnerable to external social influences (Ortmeyer, 1997; Fromm, 1930; 1941). All through his life, even through and perhaps informed by his immigration to the US, he continued to elaborate on the ways in which social structures affect and impose on the individual, and he found intellectual companionship with other psychoanalysts who shared his interpersonal and social focus and interest. In this case, the trauma of immigration was partially dealt with by focusing on how the new environment allowed for the fulfillment of an intellectual quest and a career (and a life) that was certainly endangered in Fromm's original context (country).

The view of the United States as a source of safety and professional opportunity has been described by Peter B. Neubauer (1986), an Austrian-born child psychiatrist and psychoanalyst who trained in Vienna and Bern and was influenced by Anna Freud. He arrived in the United States in 1941 and settled in New York City. Thompson (2012) quotes Neubauer, as he reflects on and eloquently verbalizes the immigrant experience:

> When I look at my experience and I hear the term "uprootedness," and if "uprootedness" refers to leaving one's own country, my immediate response is, "But I was uprooted. In Austria, in the home in which I grew up." The uprootedness was not a geographic one. The uprootedness was one of not belonging since my

childhood to the larger group. ... I did not feel uprooted leaving Vienna. I felt rather to be on the road of searching new possibilities. ... When I arrived in the United States after Switzerland and after Austria and after the uprootedness and not belonging, I had an extraordinary sense of relief, of a country which accepted me in a totally different sense than I had experienced in my childhood in Austria, in Switzerland—an openness of "Come we want you."
[cited in Thompson, 2012, p. 31, emphasis added]

It seems to me that the developmental route that psychoanalysis took in the United States emerged out of a complicated interplay between the local culture, history, and personal anxieties. The large number of refugee analysts' and their psychological needs related to their status as immigrants and to the theoretical landscape that characterized the European and American analytic scene at the time. Looking back on the origins of the interpersonal school specifically, one can see that Sullivan's and other founding members' ideas were truly novel in their intellectual content, even revolutionary at the time. These ideas emerged, even thrived, because they matched so well with some European immigrants' sensibilities. Simultaneously, the rigidifying local institutional structure rejected analysts with a cultural and social focus, inadvertently contributing to the establishment of a string of institutes centering around interpersonal ideas. The immigrants themselves on both sides of the equation seemed to have made their attachment to psychoanalysis into a psychological life-line; a source of continuity between their old-country and new immigrant selves. This was also a way to turn their eyes away from their losses. Neither the host society nor the immigrants wanted to deal with the pains of immigration, for different reasons I imagine. This reluctance and shunning of the immigrant experience manifested itself on the level of theory that was explicitly formulated as well as on the level of omitted thought that should have been articulated.

As Ricardo Ainslie and his co-authors suggest in their study of immigration among psychoanalysts, "Theorizing about immigration did not make sense in terms of the classical drive model formulations, because environment was secondary to gratification" (Ainslie et al., 2013, p. 664). Here, social conditions and environmental context were relegated "to little more than a site for the expression, redirection, and/or frustration of internal pressures" (Ainslie et al., 2013, p. 664). Accordingly, following directly from the Freudian one-person model, the assumption was advanced in classical circles that there is a single cultural and linguistic matrix shared by both patient and analyst that defines an average expectable environment (Piccioli, 2002). In this world, there was nothing to talk about when it came to immigration. The omission of a literature on immigration and of cross-cultural studies from that era, as Carola Mann (2002) points out, was much more surprising when it came to the cultural-interpersonal wing of psychoanalysis. Mann states that interpersonal psychoanalysis was particularly well-suited for addressing cultural differences and their significance; the notion of a two-person psychology and the open-ended quality of the detailed inquiry was specifically designed to do away with presumptions and assumptions like the one above, and focus on the actual, lived experience that lends itself very well to the exploration of 'the other.'

In Salman Akhtar's interpretation, the immigrants may have wanted "to forget their traumatic departures from their countries of origin, to deny cultural differences between themselves and their patients, and to become rapidly assimilated at a professional level, [so] they had no desire to draw others' (and their own) attention to their ethnic and national origins" (Akhtar, 1999, p. 23). In other words, the immigrants may have wanted to feel that they fit in, and they could do so only if they were 'not dwelling on' the past – something quite 'American,' and quite ironic for a psychoanalyst. This allowed the immigrants to stay away from pain and mourning and loss, and it allowed the host society to feel good about itself, like a savior who had done the job. American analysts could thus split off/not own up to their fear surrounding the influx of immigrants and their defensive need to control the newcomers. From an interpersonal angle, talking about the immigrant experience would have created anxiety in the 'mother' society, and thus the 'child' immigrant adapted by keeping silent, minimizing her own need to talk. And conversely, the mother society could embrace her adopted child, only as long as the adoption itself remained unspoken. An unintended consequence of the silence also emerged: "the myth of the value-free analytic endeavor [was generated], resulting in the renunciation by psychoanalysis of its cultural responsibility" (Piccioli, 2002, p. 697).

Political Backdrop as a Context and Subject

All these changes *within* the psychoanalytic scene occurred against the backdrop of the broader social-political processes that were shaping the United States and Europe at the time. The developments outlined above took place during the mid-20th century, the rise of Nazism and the World War II. The United States was instrumental in blocking the Nazi's attempts to rule the globe, and while a fear of communism began to infiltrate its institutions around the same time, social awareness and individual responsibility, empathy for others, and free exchange of ideas were still part of the mainstream conversation. Many longstanding social injustices remained, and myopic, destructive political decisions were made, of course. But an overall optimistic attitude still reigned with regard to humanity's future, mostly linked with technological advances but coupled with a genuine interest in humans themselves (Snowden, 2019). These circumstances helped psychoanalysis become one of the leading disciplines of medical sciences treating psychopathology at the time.

This overarching optimism is reflected in almost all of Weigert's writings, several of which combine phenomenological and existential philosophical considerations with psychoanalytic concepts and attitudes (Weigert, 1970, reprinted from 1949; 1962). In Weigert's opinion, it is a 'loving care' that the analyst shall provide to the patient, based on mutual trust, that in turn allows for the organization of self and ego, for the emergence of self-fulfillment and genuine self-expression, for the ability to tolerate existential anxiety and guilt, and to generate subjective order out of chaos. She considers love – based on Martin Buber's writings – the genuine ability to mutually know and care for self and other in a way that lacks possessiveness, competitiveness, and transcends each of the participants' self-centered preoccupations and anxieties. She acknowledges the difficulty inherent in all human relationships, what Sullivan was so keyed into, but she seemed to have maintained a very positive view of human nature and development. Her empathy, profound hope, and belief in psychoanalysis contributed without a doubt to her remarkable success with the severely mentally ill. In the personal sphere, her intellectual focus and optimism seemed to have also derived from a deep self-affirming need to believe that she was able to help others, since she grew up with two quite severely ill parents and had several intense depressive episodes of her own.

In the decades of the 1950s and 1960s, analysts were generally revered, their ideas were taken seriously, and they made a predictably good living. America's standing in the world was similarly high; other countries looked to it for direction, and its positive legacy from its participation in WWII was still lingering. With the Cold War, however, the US was pulled further to the right – probably as a direct result of having to represent the polar opposite of communism and the Soviet Union, as the world was splitting into an ideological duality. As an overall trend, especially since the 1980s when the US emerged victorious from these battles, the country experienced a significant, dramatic shift towards an idealization of power steeped in material success. Efficiency and 'freedom' became of primary concerns, and self-interest and competitiveness came to be the guiding value for most. Left-leaning efforts that used to drive large-scale government programs in the earlier 20th century were now labeled socialist and were rejected by large sections of the population; consumerism and greed forced greater and greater efficiency and exploitation; prejudice, racism, anti-immigrant sentiments became flagrant yet again, especially since the tragedy of the attacks on September 11, 2001. Internationally, the global benevolence of the United States was called into question; many countries see it now as self-interested and as engaging in economic colonization. In the past four years, of course, the United States' narcissistic attitude and inability to be a team player, let alone to be a trusted leader, became obvious – while its right-wing preoccupations and methods are echoed and supported by a global trend in the rise of right-wing governments.

This movement towards the political right, towards self-interest, and towards a desire for efficiency, control, simplicity – and essentially a splitting off of connectedness, vulnerability, and inclusiveness, may be an inevitability that was slowly approaching. A general disappointment took over after the hopefulness of mid-century America (Snowden, 2019), and hardship, loss of power and status, coupled with a nostalgia for, and an idealization of, the 'good old times' was going to generate a narcissistic and externalizing response. These qualities that now come to the fore need to be faced and re-integrated into America's self-image. It is in this context that psychoanalysis came to be seen as having failed to live up to the expectations in terms of providing clear solutions, efficient treatments, and answers. Psychoanalysis is portrayed now as the epitome of inefficiency, obscurity, and the unscientific remnant of the past. There is a widening gap between the mainstream cultural values and behaviors on the one hand, and what psychoanalysis holds true and has to offer on the other. One could say that while in the decades of the 1950s and 1960s, the strength and power of medicine and psychoanalysis in the United States pushed forward the assimilation of immigrants, lifting them into the ongoing mainstream discourse, our current climate turns all of us psychoanalysts into immigrants in this country, immigrants who now cannot even assimilate without losing their (our) identity entirely.

This is not necessarily the case in other countries, where psychoanalysis has been less medicalized, and thus held not to the simplistic standard of providing a cure, but more to the standard of rigorous thought and creative new ideas, situated in the interdisciplinary between hard sciences, social sciences, philosophy, and the arts (Chrzanowski, 1977). In my opinion, in the United States, Brill and subsequent analysts advocating for medicalization helped psychoanalysis to become respected and accepted in the short run but at the cost of splitting off psychoanalysis' philosophical, artistic, mystical roots/qualities, the same way the immigrants' loss of Europe was split off as part of the process of acculturation – the loss of a Europe that was culturally diverse, prone to tangents, and had the history of generating more questions than answers. European psychoanalysts, starting with Freud himself, always had apprehensions about what psychoanalysis would become in the pragmatic climate of the United States, feeling vindicated by the rise of ego-psychology (see, e.g., Lacan, 2002). I think these concerns about psychoanalysis are misguided to the degree that they assume that psychoanalysis can ultimately be controlled and restricted. In my opinion, psychoanalysis' strength lies precisely in the fact that any pressure and expectation imposed upon it by society automatically generate its own resistance and serves as a source of reflection and subversion, 'new grist for the mill' with the possibility of moving analytic theorizing and practice further. For example, as we saw before, the dominance of ego-psychology eventually and inadvertently contributed to the formation and solidification of a whole new cultural division within psychoanalysis.

So, psychoanalysis cannot be reduced to a branch of medical science without denying its interdisciplinary parts and interests – as Chrzanowski (1977) put it: it is "a hybrid between philosophy, theology, psychology and medicine" (p. 176). It has a lot to say about mental health, indeed, but always in relation to societal health and processes, by participating in public intellectual discourse, situating all of its questions within existential considerations. From this vantage point, the quick assimilation to American pragmatism and the suppression of more European sensibilities within psychoanalysis that favor uncertainty, ambiguity, and the un-resolvability of dilemmas created the temporary impression at the time that psychoanalysis had a place and could (should?) snugly fit in into American society. American society at the time also wanted psychoanalysis to fit in and come to benefit the public in tangible ways. Weigert's and her contemporaries' optimism expressed a partial, simplified objective for our discipline and was reinforced by their own personal needs and defenses as well as the cultural restriction of those times. Today, though, it is not only that society moved to a direction that undermined the type of fitting in that psychoanalysis may have been capable of in a different era, but the split-off aspects of the discipline were, I believe, destined to return, ensuring that psychoanalysis ends up on the fringes, on the margins (as a 'marginal product' from the unconscious) anyway, as it is obliged to be by its true nature. Psychoanalysis is always an unexpected, a newcomer from a distant land, far from our consciousness, a bearer of bad news; it is always looking to articulate and describe what society wants to hide or turn a blind eye to. Its cure consists in bringing into and bearing in consciousness precisely what is uncurable – and if we do a good job, we are never welcome, but peoples' minds and the social environment do change.

In order to do a good job, I think we have to accept our mission and our misfitted hybrid nature to its fullest; we have to choose being on the fringes because we actually belong there! The right-wing and ego-centric shift in the broader society that took place recently may have placed us back in a position that is actually pregnant with possibilities if we use it to reconnect ourselves with our strength. We are thus freed from the pressure – and possibility – to assimilate and fit

in. Further, to echo Carola Mann's sentiment from earlier, the interpersonal school may have an advantage in dealing with such a predicament. Its ability to bridge the intrapsychic with the external; its
history with political and social scientific ideas; its very own hybrid
and marginal origins that understood health and pathology as con-
textual from the beginning, may serve as a guide to turn this current situation to our advantage. Interpersonal psychoanalysis is well
equipped to relate the individual's desires and struggles to issues such
as systemic and individual racial discrimination; the consequences
of 'wild capitalism' and profound societal inequality for all of us; the
existential threat intertwined with a sense of dependence felt in relation to immigrants and minorities; and other currently salient concerns that are in the forefront of peoples' minds. One must add, of
course, that conversely, unless we interpersonalists do address psychic functioning in light of societal concerns and keep acknowledging the impact of the 'actual' on the 'psychological,' and unless we
can embrace our hybrid roots, we will lose our distinctive feature and
identity and probably our entire discipline will truly become obsolete. As Gerard Chrzanowski (1977) put it, "psychoanalysis has been
increasingly integrated into many socio-economic and political currents of our time. [...] Psychoanalysis is a cultural manifestation, and
accordingly must deal with the interplay of particulars within the cultural climate that prevails" (p. 176).

The Contingent Person and the Existential
Choice of Becoming a Psychoanalyst

This reflection on the changing times, on the historical roots and
current position of psychoanalysis, and on the question of identity,
these all bring us to one of the most important aspects of the human
condition: that modern man – as Ágnes Heller puts it – is a 'contingent person.' Ágnes Heller, a friend of my family, was a Hungarian
neo-Marxist existential philosopher, member of the Budapest School,
and early student of Gyorgy Lukacs. She was an immigrant herself,
spending time first in Australia and then 25 years on the faculty of
the New School in New York, until finally she returned to Hungary
in the last years of her life to confront the right-wing political realities there. Heller was always interrogating the relationship between

society, culture, and the individual; she developed the concept of the 'contingent person' in her now well-known paper written in the late 1980s entitled "The contingent person and the existential choice" (1989–1990). She starts out by saying that we all are born with a particular kind of contingency: the time, location, class, social conditions that we are 'thrown into' have nothing to do with our genetic make-up or who we are as people. Pre-modern men and women were not aware of their contingency 'because blood ties and domicile were considered the determinants of human existence' (p. 55). In contrast, modern man does not receive a destination, a telos at birth: modern man is born as a cluster of possibilities without a telos – so not only has he to make a decision about his life within a given framework, but he has to choose the framework itself to make meaning out of his life. He is acutely aware of his contingency, sometimes to the detriment of making a choice. This choice is termed 'existential' because modern man has to choose him/herself. If s/he doesn't, others will choose for him; the modern predicament is one where choices need to be and will be made. If others choose for him, modern man never realizes his possibilities that s/he was born with, but his contingency remains throughout his life: "he dies without having ever truly lived" (p. 56). In this way, Heller explains that at birth we are thrown into a very specific type of freedom that is felt as 'nothing' in a triple sense: (1) there are no handrails and guidelines for how we are to be; (2) unless we choose ourselves, we remain nothing; and (3) in a related, Hegelian sense, we are born into nothing in order to become something through our choices.

In order to choose oneself, paradoxically, man has to choose intentionally what he had not chosen in the first place: to be alive, and to be alive in a modern predicament with specific contingencies. Only if he chooses to accept these givens will he be able to actually free oneself from them, because his 'contingency turns into destiny' and life turns into his "dearest property" that he is responsible for (p. 56). Existential choice forces us to be aware of and to choose to accept our *actuality* in order to be able to actively engage with it and thereby become an actual living human being ourselves. Acceptance does not equal liking, and it does not mean passive submission, either; it means that we come to accept our predicament out of our own volition not simply as a constraint on our lives, but as the very substance of our lives that we then 'work on,' that we give meaning to through 'living it' personally. We take on our contingency, the randomness that resulted in us as a potential, and turn it into our destiny and subjectivity through our choices. The existential choice is not to be confused with being a 'self-made man' or with setting goals for one's life (Heller, 1989–1990, p. 58). It is a choice of self through a choice of a particular kind of existence. The existential choice is thus irrevocable; if we tried to revoke it, our entire self crumbles. Because it is irrevocable, it generates a telos, a destiny. Further, the existential choice is inextricably intertwined with *activity* because it is through activity that we become ourselves, an activity that is for its own sake (or only to define the self) and not for reaching any specific result. Our self is not determined by the outcome, but by the commitment and the effort that we invest into the activity. This means not only that we exist only through such activity, but that we do not exist prior to such activity and we certainly do not know ourselves to be who we are without such activity (p. 58).

So if "modern man" is nothing without an existential choice, does it follow that every one of us has to and does make such a choice? It may appear so, but it is not the case. To make an existential choice, to define oneself through one's actions, is a choice itself to be made. In Heller's formulation (1989–1990), the psychoanalyst is "a person who creates the conditions for another person to choose herself" – and she adds: "And if the person does not choose, the analyst reached the limits of his power and can do no more" (p. 61). If a person fails to choose himself, his choices in life remain revocable, always open to questioning and unmoored from meaning; the goals don't bring the expected satisfaction, and the result is that one stands outside of his or her own life. Conversely, if one does make an existential choice, the consequences will affect the totality of one's self, a self that comes into being through choice. It is a very vulnerable position to be in, and yet even in its tragic possibilities, it is never disconnected from personal meaning.

Thinking about early interpersonalists, it seems to me that for most of them, becoming a psychoanalyst was such an existential choice. How to be a psychoanalyst, what that means in any given historical and societal context is to be 'figured out' (though the contingencies), and they ceaselessly engaged in this 'figuring out' process. I wonder if this is the other side of the personal investment and the resulting combativeness around theories and professional allegiances: as much as they serve a defensive and protective function (see again Eisold, 1994), they also express an investment in living – and living in a particular way. Maybe psychoanalysis itself could and had to serve as the medium to preserve the continuity of self for European émigrés, because their selves were coming into being through practicing and thinking their profession. Psychoanalysis certainly does not seem to have been 'just a job,' a means to an end, for any of them. Insofar as the psychoanalyst helps clarify the conditions for another to choose themselves, one assumes that he himself needs to make that choice for himself in the first place.

In thinking about the convergence between Heller's concepts and interpersonal psychoanalytic work, I find that there is a possibility of mutual expansion of thought. On the one hand, learning from clinical experience, the contingency of man could be extended beyond the socio-economic and historical-societal factors to include the psychological-familial predicament that one is born into. Not only because we are aware of trans-generational trauma, but also because everything that exists in the present moment on the societal scale is lived, expressed, and transmitted to us through interpersonal interactions; the present moment also comes to us already processed and experienced by the people around us. While Heller emphasizes the individual's autonomy, possibility, and responsibility to choose and own his own life, destiny, and self in relation to others, the interpersonal school highlights the ways in which this is a very complicated and delicate process. The interpersonal way of helping a patient choose herself is to own our own analytic efforts and choices as such – as ours – which in turn creates room for the patient to come to see hers as hers. Outside the consulting room, the conditions for such emotional work are often less favorable, which is why the patient comes to us in the first place. It is a process in itself to arrive at the realization (helped along by symptoms in many cases) that one has not yet chosen oneself; that one's activities remain irrelevant in some sense to his or her own existence.

Coming to make an existential choice is thus not a discrete choice, but an ongoing work and process in and of itself. This process, I believe, is re-created in each and every session when the patient is thrown into the 'nothingness,' the space within the frame – and the analyst's silent waiting. The patient has to become able to 'use' the session, which requires a commitment to articulating his own experience. The patient cannot just 'fill up' the space that is provided for this but has to own the responsibility to do something genuine with it. In this way, each time the patient – together with the analyst – creates something, s/he gets closer to creating something in his/her own life. The analyst (and the frame) is both a facilitating environment and a participant, engaging with the patient's process. The frame, accordingly, is an additional contingency of its own for the patient's process. As the patient gets actively, emotionally involved in analysis through the *activity* of articulation, he simultaneously becomes more capable and willing to make an existential choice and being involved in his life more broadly.

So, while our usual psychoanalytic conceptualizations may offer something to Heller's thought, the reverse is also true: Heller's formulation offers an opportunity to expand on interpersonal thought. Her emphasis on activity, namely, that it is activity through which we make our existential choice and become ourselves – in other words, that the self does not exist outside of its activity – shifts us away from the traditionally held centrality of insight and reflection in the analytic process. Her framework does not only highlight the importance of participation in relation to observation – which already was Sullivan's dramatic, even revolutionary, departure from the understanding of the classical analytic stance, concluding in the two-person model – it outrightly re-frames our analytic stance as primarily doing/participating, and only secondarily, as a subcategory of that, observing. Analytic theory already established that there is no possibility of not acting/actively participating in any interpersonal situation; inaction is a form of action. This is one of the main points recently highlighted on the collective level when we finally openly consider all forms of participation, passive or active, in structural racism and sexism. But Heller goes beyond dissecting the specific nature of our ongoing participation; she further adds that what matters is not just how we act, but rather the relationship of the action to the self, as mutually determining – or as detached from each other. Not making our own choice, remaining a bystander, not investing in one value or another may contribute to structural injustices and societal issues, but it also jeopardizes our self as a psychoanalyst as well as the future of our discipline.

Unless we grapple with our current societal predicament (contingency), unless we recognize it as personal and meaningful, and unless we engage in activity that itself amounts to an existential choice, we will not stand for what we believe, and thus we cannot believe in what we allegedly stand for. We do become obsolete for the present-day society and the collective consciousness of our times, and psychoanalysis becomes obsolete for us personally, in our lives. This suggestion is, in my understanding, a departure from the simply construed 'neutral' or value-free analytic stance. More broadly, though, interpersonal psychoanalysis has a quite clear ethical foundation: a profound respect for 'others" experience as equally valid to one's own; an acknowledgment that through our participation, we always bear some responsibility for whatever unfolds in an interaction, and finally, that *actual interaction, actuality*, plays a central role in experience, which we seek to see, observe, reflect on, and openly talk about.

References

Ainslie, R.C., Harlem, A., Tummala-Narra, P., Barbanel, L., and Ruth, R. (2013). Contemporary psychoanalytic views on the experience of Immigration. *Psychoanalytic Psychology*, 30, 663–679.

Akhtar, S. (1999). The immigrant, the exile, and the experience of nostalgia. *Journal of Applied Psychoanalytic Studies*, 1, 123–130.

Antokoletz, J.C. (1994). Cross-cultural passages. *The American Journal of Psychoanalysis*, 54, 279–281.

Bryce, A. (2020). A history of the Washington Baltimore Center for Psychoanalysis. *The International Journal of Controversial Discussion*, 2, 174–180.

Burnham, D. (1978). Orthodoxy and eclecticism in American psychoanalysis: The Washington-Baltimore experience. In J. Quen and E. Carlson (Eds.) *American Psychoanalysis: Origins and Development*. New York: Brunner Mazel, pp. 87–108.

Chrzanowski, G. (1977). Some present day psychoanalytic currents on the European continent. *Journal of American Academy of Psychoanalysis and Dynamic Psychiatry*, 5, 175–178.

Eisold, K. (1994). The intolerance of diversity in psychoanalytic institutions. *International Journal of Psychoanalysis*, 75, 785–800.

Fromm, E. (1930). *The Working Class of Weimar Germany*, trans. B. Weinberger. Cambridge, MA: Harvard University Press, 1984.

Fromm, E. (1941). *Escape from Freedom*. New York: Rinehart & Co, pp. 305

Heller, Á. (1989–1990). The contingent person and the existential choice. *The Philosophical Forum*, XXI:1–2, 53–69.

Holmes, M. (2010). Dusseldorf-Berlin-Ankara-Washington. *Psychiatry*, 73:1, 1–33.

Lacan, J. (2002). The function and field of speech and language in psychoanalysis. In *Ecrits*, trans.B. Fink, New York, London: W.W. Norton & Company, pp. 197–268.

Mann, C. (2002). Cross-cultural psychoanalysis and the interpersonal perspective. *International Forum of Psychoanalysis*, 11, 309–312.

Neubauer, P. (1986). Panel: The experience of migration. Oral History Workshop 25, Archives, American Psychoanalytic Association, Oskar Diethelm Library, Weill Cornell Medical College.

Ortmeyer, D.H. (1997). Revisiting our psychoanalytic toots. *Contemporary Psychoanalysis*, 33, 313–322.

Osman, M.P. (2004). The role of an early-life variant of the Oedipus complex in motivating religious endeavors. *Journal of the American Psychoanalytic Association*, 52, 975–997.

Parens, H. (2001). On society's crimes against itself. *Journal of Applied Psychoanalytic Studies*, 3, 221–229.

Piccioli, E. (2002). IPA Congress summary of the panel of Psychoanalysis Across Cultural and Linguistic Difference: Conceptual and Technical Issues. *International Journal of Psychoanalysis*, 83, 695–701.

Ponder, J. (2007). Elitism in psychoanalysis in the USA: Narcissistic defense against cumulative traumas of prejudice and exclusion. *International Journal of Applied Psychoanalytic Studies*, 4, 15–30.

Richards, A. (2006). Creating sociology and psychoanalysis in the Habsburg Lands: Freud, Brill, and Fleck. Presented at the 50th Annual Leo Baeck Memorial Address.

Shapiro, S. (2017). The history of the William Alanson White Institute sixty years after Thompson. *Contemporary Psychoanalysis*, 53, 44–62.

Snowden, F.M. (2019). *Epidemics and Society: From the Black Death to the Present*. New Haven and London: Yale University Press, p. 582.

Thompson, N.L. (2012). The transformation of psychoanalysis in America: Emigré analysts and the New York Psychoanalytic Society and Institute, 1935–1961. *Journal of the American Psychoanalytic Association*, 60, 9–44.

Weigert-Vowinkel, E. (1938). The cult and mythology of the Magna Mater from the standpoint of psychoanalysis. *Psychiatry: Journal of the Biology and the Pathology of Interpersonal Relations*, 1, 347–378.

Weigert, E. (1970). *The Courage to Love: Selected Papers of Edith Weigert, M.D.* New Haven and London: Yale University Press, p. 408.

William Alanson White Psychiatric Foundation (1938). Mission statement. *Psychiatry: Journal of the Biology and the Pathology of Interpersonal Relations*, 1, ii.

Chapter 8

Considering the Radical Contributions of Clara Mabel Thompson

Ann D'Ercole

The life of Clara Mabel Thompson (1893–1958), a 20th century pioneering psychoanalyst, is inspiring, and yet her achievements have been underappreciated. One could look no further than her groundbreaking essay, "Notes on the Psychoanalytic Significance of the Choice of Analyst" (1938), to understand how she changed the field of psychoanalysis. The essay, written five years after the death of her second analyst, her mentor and collaborator Sándor Ferenczi, boldly introduces the concept of a two-person encounter in the analytic situation. With Harry Stack Sullivan's invitation to publish in the inaugural issue of *Psychiatry*, Thompson skillfully shifts the focus from trying to understand the mind of the patient, to discovering the continuous dynamic relationship between the analyst and analysand. It marks the introduction of the reciprocity of the psychoanalytic encounter, the continuous mutually influencing character of psychoanalytic therapy. This relationship, she points out, can begin even before the prospective couple meets. In 1938, those words must have been shocking. Her radical perspective challenged existing psychoanalytic conceptions of the role of the analyst as detached and objective. Instead, she offered a view of the analyst as possessing utterly human qualities and shortcomings. She broadened the field of psychoanalysis to include the social-cultural context.

While Freud was interested in society, it was chiefly as a world whose group processes reflected individual dynamics and to an extent restructured them and passed them down in the structures of guilt and conscience (D'Ercole, 2017). Thompson introduced a new psychoanalysis—an American brand[1], more mutual, egalitarian,

DOI: 10.4324/9781003270355-9

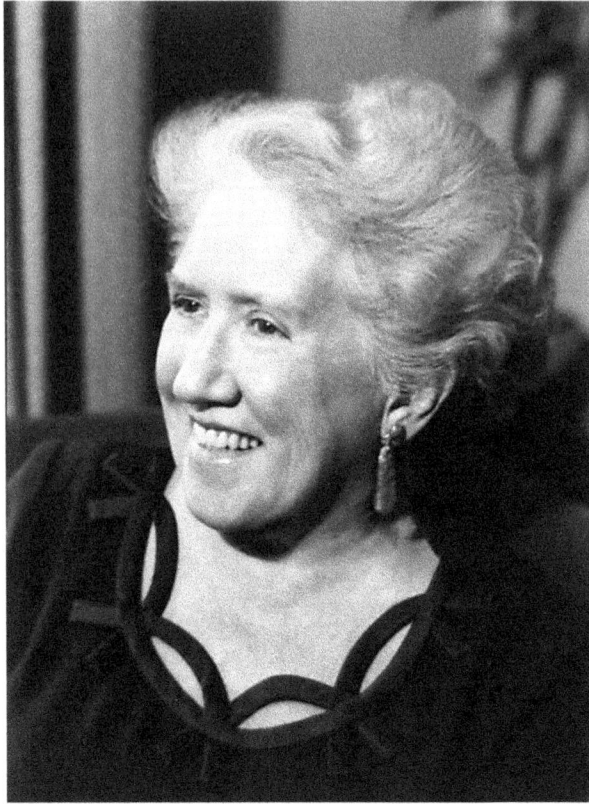

Figure 8 Clara Thompson, 1950, Gado Images/Alamy Stock Photo.

and focused on the analyst-patient relationship. By the 1940s, Thompson was also contributing groundbreaking essays on the psychology of women. While Karen Horney (1939) offered cultural critiques of Freud's theories about women, she eventually turned her attention elsewhere; Thompson became the "standard-bearer" for a cultural understanding of the psychology of women (Capelle, 1993, p. 14).

Yet, Clara Thompson is overlooked, both for her contributions to the development of the Interpersonal/Relational tradition in psychoanalysis and for her contributions to the psychology of women. How do we understand this omission? Does it have to do with gender in a patriarchal profession? Or is it the result of the field's history of silencing dissenting voices: a "death by silence," as Menaker

(1989) and Rachman (2018) have described? Whatever the cause, the time has come for a course correction. It is time to acknowledge how Clara Thompson established an American psychoanalytic tradition.

Who is Clara Thompson? She was a daring woman who entered psychoanalysis on the ground floor. She was a scholar, a teacher, a leader, and the director of a psychoanalytic training institute where she mentored dozens of eminent psychoanalysts. Her scholarship includes over 40 essays and reviews. Her book, *Psychoanalysis: Evolution and Development* (1950c), is a tour de force that grew from students' requests for copies of her lectures at various schools and institutes, including Johns Hopkins Medical School, New York Medical College, New York Psychoanalytic Institute, New School for Social Research, Washington School of Psychiatry, and the William Alanson White Institute of Psychiatry.

The Person, the Context, and the Theory

Understanding the contributions of Clara Thompson is enhanced by knowing Clara Thompson the person—to whatever degree we can know someone. The way she was raised and educated, the way she rebelled, and how she flourished and was constricted, is all part of the wide-ranging story of her life (D'Ercole, in press). Thompson became a "modern woman"– an early 20th century term for women who challenged gender conformity.

Theories reflect the people who create them. Thompson was thoughtful, empathic, and respectful of others. Those characteristics informed her clinical work. She was uncommonly forthright and profoundly clear in her approach to theory. As she said to a friend, "I couldn't become complicated if I tried" (Green, 1964, p. 375). Thompson was an outspoken advocate of a new psychoanalysis following her own transformative therapeutic experience as both a patient and a therapist working with Sándor Ferenczi. She was aware of how changing social conditions led to different ways of knowing. As a feminist, she fully believed in equality. That belief in many ways structured her life and is inherent in her clinical theories and practices.

Thompson was born in 1893 in Providence, Rhode Island, an important and active hub for commerce. The Thompson family were members of the Free Will Baptist Church. As a child, Thompson, who was called Mabel by her family, was active and engaged with her peers. She was liked, and she wanted to please. Her very religious mother was harsh, righteous, and rigid; her father was warm and ambitious, and she adored him. We know these historical details primarily from Maurice Green, a former student who wrote an informative biographical essay that he tucked into an edited volume of her collected papers, *Interpersonal Psychoanalysis: The Selected Papers of Clara M.* Thompson (1964).

Thompson's parents, Frank and Clara, were given a large house on their marriage. Her grandparents had hopes of lots of grandchildren, perhaps, but Thompson had only one sibling, Frank, seven years younger and his mother's favorite. By then, an extended family of grandparents, aunts, and uncles were living under one roof. One side of the family, the maternal side, were strict followers of the tenants of the Free Will Baptist church, while the paternal side, also Free Will Baptists, were less observant. The Free Will Baptists accepted the Bible as the word of God; they believed in self-governance and rejected the Puritan movement on the grounds that the Puritan's belief—God will provide—led to a lack of social mobility. In contrast, the Free Will Baptists believed the Bible, as God's inspiration, should be believed, obeyed, and not altered. They also believed that everyone sins and needs salvation. For Free Will Baptists, the "choice" to repent for one's sins represented freedom. Ultimately, faith was the condition of salvation, therefore spreading the faith was critical. For women, there were rigid social requirements of self-sacrifice and self-denial. As an adolescent, Clara Thompson wanted to become a medical missionary; she would join the Free Will Baptist Woman's Missionary Society, one of the few options available to women outside of marriage that seemed to offer a chance for adventure as they traveled the world to save souls. Pleasing her mother was certainly part of those youthful aspirations. Of importance in the discussion of the Free Will Baptists and Thompson's legacy is that they were strong abolitionists, an influence that can be heard in her later writing.

Clara Thompson's allegiances changed at Pembroke College/Brown University,[2] where she was exposed to a different group of people with distinctly different ideas. For example, in college, she read *Mill on the Floss* (Eliot, 1860), where she identified with the protagonist

Maggie's desire for a larger life. Thompson's identification with Maggie exposed her conflict between her desire for a fuller life of love and adventure versus her allegiance to a missionary's pledge of virtuous deprivation and self-denial. This struggle contributed to her growing unhappiness.

During this period, she stopped attending church, causing a rupture with her mother to whom she did not speak for decades, though they reconciled later in her life. Thompson also refused a marriage proposal from a major in the United States medical corps because he demanded she abandon her plans for a career in medicine. She was troubled by her decision but held firm to her career goal, graduating from Johns Hopkins School of Medicine in 1920, the year white women gained the right to vote. By then, Thompson had met other women who were interested in medicine; one in particular, Lucile Dooley, had a PhD in psychology and was already working in a psychiatric hospital. Thompson decided to pursue psychiatry. She worked under Adolf Meyer, William Alanson White, and in her second year of residency in 1923, she became friends with Harry Stack Sullivan.

Thompson had discovered Freud's writings as a young medical school resident immersing herself in the early books and ideas in the field, and she was an enthusiastic learner. At the time, the field of psychoanalysis itself was about twenty years old. She described it in the following way:

> The workers in the earlier years concentrated on finding more effective methods of therapy and on trying to enlarge the therapeutic scope of psychoanalysis. There was a shift in emphasis from concern with recall of the past (the removal of the infantile amnesia) to the understanding of the dynamics of the doctor-patient relationship as observed in treatment. This interest did not disappear after 1934; it became embodied in Sullivan's theory of interpersonal relations. Increased study of comparative culture in the later 1920s eventually contributed significantly to another challenging of Freud's biological theory of neurosis by the so-called cultural school of analysts, whose thinking began to influence psychoanalysis around 1934.
>
> (Thompson, 1950c, p. 5)

In her 1950s book, she identifies the clinical discoveries of Rank and Ferenczi who moved away from Freud's notion of recovering childhood "amnesia" and instead promoted the idea that the patient was not suffering so much from the past but from the way the past was influencing present-day behaviors (Thompson, 1950c, p. 14).

The Enduring Connections of Thompson, Ferenczi, Horney, Sullivan, and Fromm

"Notes on the Psychoanalytic Significance of the Choice of Analyst" (Thompson, 1938) introduces an interdisciplinary model of therapy influenced not only by Thompson's work with Ferenczi but also by anthropologists and other social scientists. By 1929, Edward Sapir, Harry Stack Sullivan, and William Alanson White were at work contributing to this interdisciplinary model (Wake, 2011). This group is important in the history of interpersonal psychoanalysis; their ideas preceded the publication of the journal *Psychiatry* and Thompson's essay by ten years.

Thompson's relationship with Sullivan was of particular significance. They met during her residency when she was giving a paper on schizophrenia. Sullivan was drawn to her because of her interest in the topic and because she seemed ill. He thought she might be schizophrenic, but in fact, she had typhoid. They took to each other immediately and were close friends for life. They were both interested in the work of Sándor Ferenczi. After attending a lecture by Sándor Ferenczi, Thompson asked Ferenczi if he would become her analyst. Having no time available on his visit to New York, Ferenczi encouraged her to come to Budapest for treatment; she was startled by the invitation but accepted. Imagine traveling across an ocean for therapy.

Thompson (1988) was in treatment with Ferenczi in Budapest from 1928 to 1933, and she explored similar ideas to those of Sullivan and other American culturalists.[3] When she told Ferenczi that his thinking was in line with what she and Sullivan were discussing, he gently accused her of stealing his ideas: "He could not believe that Sullivan had developed a way of thinking that was so close to his own, without any collaboration" (Thompson, 2017, p. 8).[4] What Thompson herself does not acknowledge at that moment is that she was a collaborating link between Ferenczi and Sullivan. By 1943, she proclaimed in her essay 'The Therapeutic Technique of Sándor Ferenczi': "I am a pupil of Ferenczi and for over ten years I have made use of some of his techniques in my psycho-analytic work. In the course of time I have discarded several of his ideas and confirmed the validity of others" (1943a, p. 64).

While Thompson was Ferenczi's disciple, she was not a blind admirer. She had been taught at Pembroke College to not take ideas "off the counter"; instead, her teachers promoted "a skepticism about received ideas" (see discussion in Capelle, 1993, p. 152). This foundational educational experience helped to facilitate the development of Thompson's critical thinking and helped her imagine that she could live life according to her own rules.

Thompson's analysis with Ferenczi is a long and complex story that includes Ferenczi's tenderness and his "relaxation technique," where he eventually permitted Thompson to kiss him as often as she liked (see Dupont, 1988). She felt Ferenczi gave her a chance to experience a "happy childhood...I came to have relationships with people for the first time. In a comfortable social way. I still have difficulties with intimacy, although not too much" (Eissler & Thompson, 1952). Thompson left that analysis feeling changed, more open, and less isolated. There is a reference in Ferenczi's *Diary* to her as a victim of childhood sexual abuse that has been discussed by Rachman (1997), Rudnytsky (2015), and Shapiro (1993), who each take up the abuse and its sequelae. There is little doubt that Thompson was wounded in childhood, certainly by her harsh, physically abusive mother and perhaps by a sexually abusive father; in that regard, questions remain. Untangling the knot between Ferenczi's wish to safe-keep the anonymity of his patients and the blatant disclosure of Thompson's identity and discussion of her sexual abuse clouds rather than clarifies what is known.[5]

On her return from Budapest, Thompson moved to New York where her friend Sullivan was living. She was also friends with Karen Horney and Erich Fromm. From the mid to late 1930s, Thompson, Sullivan, Horney, and Fromm played together, shared ideas, and learned from each other. Their interpersonal boundaries were fluid; Fromm became Thompson's third analyst and Thompson became Sullivan's analyst. Thompson's analysis of Sullivan lasted about

300 hours and ended abruptly when she tried to tackle his pattern of overspending. Her analysis with Fromm lasted for quite some time. The correspondence between Thompson and Fromm reveals that they stayed close friends for the rest of her life.

Thompson remained friends with Horney through the early New York Psychoanalytic wars, when Horney was demoted and Thompson and colleagues left in protest (Frosch, 1991). But Thompson broke with Horney after Horney prevented Fromm from becoming a training analyst at their newly formed institute, the Association for the Advancement of Psychoanalysis, arguing, as she did, that Fromm was a "lay analyst." The situation was complicated further by the fact that Fromm and Horney had a relationship over many years that came to an end around that time (Perry, 1982; Friedman, 2013). Overall, Thompson felt that Sullivan had the most influence over her thinking for the longest period of time. And as Thompson explains, when Fromm and Horney came along, "we were very much in the same line as Sullivan" (2017, p. 19).

The Psychology of Women

Thompson's contributions to an understanding of gender in a patriarchal culture were trailblazing. Her predecessor, Karen Horney, abandoned this line of thought after the 1930s to develop a system of psychoanalytic theory and therapy that focused on individual psychological development. Thompson, on the other hand, held fast to a culturalist view of women for two decades. Take, for example, "'Penis Envy' in Women" (1943b)[6]:

> "Penis envy" is a term coined by Freud and used by him to describe a basic attitude found in neurotic women. The term had more than symbolic meaning to him. He was convinced that this envy in women grew out of a feeling of biological lack beginning with the little girl's discovery in early childhood that she lacked something possessed by the little boy...In brief, we have shown that cultural factors can explain the tendency of women to feel inferior about their sex and their consequent tendency to envy men; that this state of affairs may well lead women to blame all their difficulties on the fact of their sex...

The position of underprivilege might be symbolically expressed in the term "penis envy" using the penis as the symbol of the more privileged sex.

(pp. 123–125)

Thompson (1959), in "An Introduction to Minor Maladjustments," was the first to compare discrimination against women with racism.

Sexual difference is an obvious difference, and obvious differences are especially convenient marks of derogation in any competitive situation in which one group aims to get power over the other.

Discrimination because of color is a case in point. Here, a usually easily distinguishable difference is a sign which taken as adequate justification for gross discrimination and underprivilege. A negro should feel himself inferior because he has a black skin. Obviously, the black skin is important to the group in power because it is such an easily recognized characteristic with which to differentiate a large number of people from themselves. Everything is done to make it a symbol for all the inferiority feelings Negros have. Few indeed of the governing class can be so fatuous as to believe that black skin implies an intrinsic inferiority.

(pp. 243–244)

In her paper, "Cultural Pressures in the Psychology of Women" (1942), Thompson argues,

In my study of "The Role of Women in This Culture[7]" I presented a survey of the present status of women in the United States. I pointed out the basic situation and the changes which are going on. Although the paper was chiefly concerned with the positive aspects of woman's evolution, I spoke also to the problems still remaining, and the new problems arising in the new situations.

This is essentially a patriarchal culture and although many values are changing and these changes on the whole are working to the advantage of women, the patriarchal situation still presents limitations to a women's free development of her interests...the official attitude of the culture toward women has been and still is to the effect that woman is not the equal of man.

(p. 277)

Thompson's Role as Founder of Interpersonal Psychoanalysis

Thompson's "Notes on the Psychoanalytic Significance of the Choice of Analyst" (1938) in *Psychiatry* establishes her position as the leader in the Interpersonal tradition. Up until the introduction of *Psychiatry*, the premiere psychoanalytic journal was *The International Journal of Psychoanalysis*. In contrast, *Psychiatry*, the brain-child of Harry Stack Sullivan as founding editor, distinguished itself by not using the term "psychoanalysis." Sullivan wanted to emphasize that the journal would be exploring the spaces in between psychiatry, psychoanalysis, the social sciences, and biology. Included among the essays in the issue is one by Thompson's and Sullivan's friend, the anthropologist Ruth Benedict (1938), which addresses the strength of cultural conditioning. According to Conci (2012), this essay is "a comparative anthropological analysis of the supportive or inhibiting effect of a child's upbringing on their acceptance of their role as adults later in life" (p. 299). Also, in the issue is Lucile Dooley's "The Genesis of Psychological Sex Differences" (1938). Dooley reappears often in the life story of Clara Thompson. She was responsible for getting Thompson her first job and remained her friend throughout life, even though Dooley seems to have held onto quintessential Freudian biological determinism (see Peters, 1979). Other articles in *Psychiatry* carry an interdisciplinary imprint, including Thompson's essay, which reflects the influence of Ferenczi and is perhaps a nod to his request for her to bring his ideas back to America.

A central idea in the original interpersonal tradition is the mutually influencing and influential aspects of any interpersonal encounter, a concept originally developed by 19th century anthropologists (D'Ercole, 2017). Thompson (1950c) points out: "About 1930, a few analysts had begun to show a new kind of interest in anthropological studies of culture, and one anthropologist, Edward Sapir, was a pioneer in advocating collaboration of anthropology, sociology and psychoanalysis" (p. 194). The collaboration goes back further than Thompson indicates. In an investigation into where the concept of participant observation (often attributed to Sullivan) began, D'Ercole (2017) explains that the person who popularized the term was the anthropologist Bronislaw Malinowski (1922/2013).

But he was not the originator of the idea; that was another anthropologist, Frank Hamilton Cushing (1922/1998). Malinowski, like Cushing, actively lived with the people he was studying instead of sifting through field reports from afar or relying on single informants. Sullivan knew Malinowski and gave credit to him for the term. The blending of anthropology, sociology, and psychiatry led to the development of the so-called "life history" method, which was based on a three-part interview that combined the study of personality, the conventions of social psychiatry, and participant-observation. The scientists using this "life history" interview tried to spell out all things that could possibly influence a "person" over the course of his or her lifespan, including questions about one's social environment. These interviewers and the interviewees encountered the lived complexity of this process as they went about refining it. They discovered that the interviewer was a "participant" in the process of discovery, and that no information was devoid of the influence of both participants.

This interdisciplinary legacy forms the basis for Thompson's (1938) notion of the mutually influencing role of the analyst and patient. She argued for a social therapeutic model that steps outside of the developmental, interpretive model of therapy and begins with the choice of the analyst.

Any study of the phenomenon that appear in psychoanalysis has its difficulties. The context is prolonged over a long period, meaning often attaches to subtleties that are hard to recapture, and fully convincing explorations have usually to be admitted in the interest of the therapeutic result. There are, however, some publish data of observation that can be appraised objectively. Of this information, that pertaining to the analyst's part in the collaboration is the more glaringly inadequate. One seldom finds an account of anything that suggests the differences in personality of various psychoanalysts, or the significant entering of the analyst's personality anywhere in the whole protracted process. Many analysts, however, must have failed with some patient who did better elsewhere; must have carried to completion some patients who had failed with a preceding analyst.

Moreover, every psychoanalysis has a beginning, and patients often exercise what is called choice in selecting the person with whom they will undertake the work.

(p. 205)

Her plain-spoken and pragmatic New England style of communication can lead some to miss the significance of her remarks, but make no mistake, in 1938, Thompson is announcing a sea change in the practice of psychoanalysis. This transformation ushers in "American Psychoanalysis" and a newly developing tradition, Interpersonal Psychoanalysis. Given their close relationship, Sullivan surely knew that Thompson would be the perfect person to deliver a non-orthodox cultural view of psychoanalysis, not only because of their joint exploration of findings in anthropology and sociology, but also because Thompson's forthright, pragmatic style would allow her to bring these new ideas forward without grandstanding nor attacking others.

She delivered a view of human relationships and the analytic encounter that is not orthodox but, instead, integrates all the developing social science disciplines.

An individual has some personal reaction to every one with whom he comes in close contact and an analyst presumably is no exception in this respect. The fact, he might be expected to have some very definite feelings about someone who he expects to see daily for many months, perhaps years. While material is easily available on that rational and irrational or transference attitudes of patients, since they are important things to be investigated in every analysis, it is more difficult to observe the attitudes of the analyst and evaluate their influences on the analysis.

(p. 206)

Thompson argues that the field of inquiry in psychoanalysis is broader than that of the patient's internal world. She does not begin where Ferenczi left off by quoting him or his teachings, as she could easily have done by referencing his paper "The Elasticity of the Psychoanalytic Technique" (1928), an essay Rachman (1997) notes offers a two-person view of the analytic relationship. Rather, she uses her own individually

American voice with New England roots that are practical, unadorned, and idealistic, an outgrowth of an educational background in an ideology of liberation, using the distinctively American philosophy of Pragmatism and the life history method in psychiatry. She balances psychoanalysis with mainstream 20th century American empiricism as she talks about objectivity, observation, and data—elements of the scientific method.

Breaking Boundaries

In her 1938 article, "Notes on the Psychoanalytic Significance of the Choice of Analyst," Thompson demonstrates a willingness to go against orthodox Freudian theories stating her ideas clearly and without hesitation. It is important to note that she does this without engaging in polemical attacks. Waugaman (2016) observes that Thompson has the ability to present her ideas without the need to dismiss those who hold different opinions. It is one of her many strengths as a leader, along with an integrity that inspired others. That may also be why she qualifies her work with words that minimize rather than aggrandize. There are no grand pronouncements or empty flattery. She is a scientist at work trying to discover.

Penning cautious introductory sentences, Thompson (1938) directs attention to the role of the analyst as a whole person in the interaction with the patient, someone who brings their entire personality to doing the work. The beginning of the essay almost reads like a research paper, as she questions: What role does the analyst as an individual existing in reality play in the analytic situation? And do individual variations in the analyst have important effects for good or bad on the course of the analysis?

Thompson goes on to address her sample and methods, as she assumes each analyst is sufficiently analyzed and knows his or her issues. She accepts that a well-analyzed analyst is not infallible and maintains constant self-observation and self-criticism. She turns to the literature, citing findings about patients' attitudes about their reactions to the analyst and about transference phenomenon. She sees the flaws in the published data that present the analyst as either a fountain of detached wisdom, or a person who is not affected personally by the patient, or as someone who puts ideas into the patient's head then analyzes them out with none of it related to the patient's life—closer instead to the fantasy in the mind of the analyst. Thompson methodically dismisses each of these assumptions, giving convincing examples: "If the analyst really has no convictions on the question of stealing, can he help the patient to understand and accept the attitude of society in which the patient must live, about stealing?" (p. 206). She concludes that the notion that the analyst's attitude should be a "zero" is erroneous and impossible.

As in other places in her writing, Thompson draws from her own experience and provides autobiographical examples, sometimes identifying them as such, most times not. For example, she explains:

> Every so often one finds in reading the report of a detailed case analysis that at a certain point something in reality occurred to convince the patient of the human qualities of the analyst, e.g., some reaction to bad news received over the phone during the patient's hour, or pleasant news similarly received even some spontaneous expression of sympathy towards the patient.
>
> (p. 206)

Putting moments of authenticity, vitality, and freedom into the analytic work allows Thompson to argue that these kinds of incidents enable the patient to discard unrealistic attitudes towards the analyst and see the analyst more realistically.

In his compilation of Thompson's selected papers, Green (1964) provides an example of Thompson's engaged, spontaneous attitude.

> One day a patient was in consultation with Thompson when the phone rang. She picked up the receiver, listened to it and then hung up, saying to herself and perhaps the patient, "That bitch? That nurse Henry's got says he has cancer of the lung. He has nothing of the sort!"
>
> (p. 371)[8]

Thompson was referring to her partner Henry Major, who was ill at the time. For nearly a decade, Thompson and Major lived their unconventional life together, with Major remaining married and living in New York City during the winters while living with Thompson at her house in Provincetown in the summers. Major was a well-known artist who worked as a staff cartoonist for the Hearst papers and was renowned for his caricatures of Albert Einstein and other famous people (D'Ercole, 2017).

With a focus on the realness of the analyst and the value of a natural spontaneity, Thompson (1938) underscores the humanness of the analytic relationship.

Emotional Presence

In "Notes on the Psychoanalytic Significance of the Choice of Analyst," Thompson (1938) goes on to argue that being with a detached analyst can be a replication of a detached parent that brought the patient into treatment in the first place. Always in a conversation with her reader, she asks and answers:

> Specifically, what do people want in an analyst? They want most of all someone in whom they can have confidence, someone who makes them feel less afraid, and who they can believe knows how to cure them. This feeling of confidence has its objective and subjective origins. Actually few people are in a position to evaluate the therapeutic ability of a given analyst unless they know his work very intimately. Training reputation and experience figure in this evaluation but little else in a rational way.
>
> (p. 207)

She wisely explains how a patient's reaction to "age, cultural background, sex and personality…is only partially objective" (p. 207). Various other feelings, she warns, come into play: "the impression of strength, the feeling of the familiar, the feeling of being understood, the absence of hostile feelings either on his own part or subjectively felt as coming from the analyst make up the feeling of trust and confidence" (p. 207). These feelings include "irrational or transference factors—that is, a patient chooses in the same way that he falls in love, on the basis of his own life patterns" (p. 207).

Thompson's comparison of choosing an analyst to the way one falls in love is refreshing for its lack of jargon offering something everyone can understand. She goes on to explain that people seek out in an analyst "the person with whom they feel most capable of having an intense emotional relationship; that is, they seek the personality which most nearly corresponds to personalities with whom they tend to have attachments" (p. 208).

She warns that choosing an analyst may have the effect of reproducing in general "a parental figure or corresponding to some ideal for a love object" (p. 208). Or, conversely, many choose in a "defensive way" someone who is unlikely to fulfill negative life patterns. She gives the example of someone who chooses a man for an analyst "because the most unpleasant life problems are connected with women" (p. 208).

Thompson is a great believer in giving examples; her discussion of the fit and misfit between patients and analysts is detailed. One in particular may be autobiographical. She describes a woman who meets an analyst socially: In the course of the evening's conversation, he suggests she come into treatment with him: "Her reaction was fear but she realized that she needed analysis, that he would probably accept her for a fee which she could pay, and finally she felt irresistibly attracted to the situation" (p. 214). This could be a reference to her analytic work with her first therapist, Joseph "Snake" Thompson[9], while she was a resident. Thompson reports:

> Analysis was begun, fear continued, sleeplessness developed, difficulty in working appeared, and the patient finally lost her job... The patient in question had a neurotic attachment to her employer which was reciprocated by the employer, who also had a neurotic need for power. When this situation began to be analyzed, the analyst's jealousy reinforced the patient's own tendency to make indirect aggressions of a serious nature against her employer with disastrous consequences. Although the patient continued in analysis for some months after the loss of her position, she made no further progress, having lost confidence in the analyst on a reality basis. Later her analysis was successfully completed by another.
> (p. 214)[10]

She notes that patients in search of an analyst have their preferences. The most often discussed characteristic is the sex of the analyst. She finds that sex is only an obvious distinction and cautions that psychologically the distinction does not always hold up. She gives the example of two women being analyzed by women analysts where one says to the other, "Why on earth did you go to a woman? I wouldn't dream of being analyzed by a woman" (p. 209). The friend bursts out laughing, bringing her friend to her senses and the realization that she was after all in analysis with a woman. Since her analyst felt so much like her father, she succeeded in ignoring the actual sex of her analyst.

The Role of Interest and Empathy

Of the many observations Thompson (1938) makes, one that has not received enough attention has to do with the potency of the level of interest the analyst shows to a prospective patient. Attention to, and interest in, the patient is effective from the very beginning of their relationship. Comparing the analytic relationship to interpersonal intimacies in general, she identifies the personality of the analyst as the most important factor in the choice. That said, she also adds, "it is also the vaguest, most difficult to evaluate clearly, and is, therefore an excellent field for errors in objectivity, especially when such an error fits into the neurotic pattern of the patient" (p. 211). She observes how many analyses fail:

> One finds also another group who have to be submissive and who cannot assert themselves, even for the sake of their own self-preservation; these are also masochistic. The first group with unconscious genius finds the analyst whose specific liabilities are especially bad for them and hurl themselves to their destruction. The second group enters the analytic situation fearing that a mistake has been made, but when they find their fears confirmed and evidence accumulates that the analysis is either doing no good or actual harm in their lives they are unable to leave. They are afraid of the anger of the analyst, or they fear hurting his feelings or they fear ridicule.
>
> (p. 213)

Waugaman (2016) has noted how Thompson was ahead of her time in her analysis of certain high-risk analytic dyads, as she identifies risk factors for boundary violations: "some bad analytic situations (sic) occur when the analyst is anxious about a physically illness;

or is facing the illness or death of a loved one; or is under financial strain" (p. 16). Her observation about potential risks has since become accepted knowledge and discussed in the literature by many (e.g., Gabbard, 2016).

Beyond Reciprocity

For Thompson and those who followed her, the analyst was understood as a real person within the analytic situation. She dismissed the idea of absolute neutrality and uncorrupted transference. Also, she did not place the analyst in an exalted position above the patient. Rather, even if viewed as asymmetrical to each other, she saw each having a "highly significant" role in the process (Thompson, 1938, p. 215). Her perspective in early analytic history helped us to grapple with the dynamic relationship between analysand and psychoanalyst. This view can be heard in Levenson's (2009) edict, "one cannot *not* interact, one cannot *not* influence" (p. 172) and Stern's (1996) claim that

> the analyst had no choice but to be a real person in the treatment situation, and in the patient's experience, and that absolute neutrality and an "uncontaminated" transference therefore made no sense. The actual person of the analyst, that is, directly influenced the patient's experience.
>
> (p. 281)

Thinking of Thompson, Levenson found that after her death, she "just disappeared" from the official canon (ref.), though it is clear from the work of many contemporary luminaries, such as Stern quoted above, that her ideas are very much "in the air." Her disappearance from the canon is nonetheless a great loss.

Thompson's Relevance Today: On Race

Thompson initiated efforts to conceptualize social issues in the field of psychoanalysis. But she did not have the benefit of conceptual tools like "systemic racism" available today. We might thus understand her attempts as bold, but far from complete. They are first steps within the cultural and conceptual frame in which she was working at the time. She undertook a cultural analysis of racism, sexism, and homo-phobia at the beginning of the 20th century that explored and resisted the underlying tendency to pathologize and marginalize. At the same time, we need to examine Thompson's thinking in terms of current formulations of white privilege, a position from which she spoke and was to a large extent unaware. Even as Thompson took important steps towards liberalization, her white privilege could not but limit her analysis.

Breaking from standard disciplinary boundaries, Thompson spoke un-self-consciously to issues of social and political concern. She wrote about race, homosexuality, and the psychology of women from the perspective of women's oppression (see Thompson, 1942; 1950a; 1950b). To her credit, in her essay "Dynamics of Hostility" (Weiss et al., 1959), she speaks of race in a way that was rare in psy-choanalysis in the mid-20th century:

> If one lives constantly in an unfriendly environment, as in the case of the American Negro, it is normal to show a chronic hos-tility toward one's persecutors. These, I believe cannot be consid-ered destructive drives; they are a part of man's expression of his right and wish to live.
>
> (p. 11)

Thompson can be seen as normalizing "black anger" and can be crit-icized on a couple of counts. First, her assessment maintains a rather benevolent superiority, and second, it fails to recognize that "black anger" or "black rage" is not only as a response to persecution but also from a white stance it can be a perception, disowned from the actual reality of white rage.

Her abolitionist heritage was ensconced in the complicated entan-glements of a racist society. We can hear Thompson struggle to hold onto a nascent field theory in her analysis as she weaves in and out of individual psychological concepts that are in themselves racist:

> However, all of these emotions can become expressions of irra-tional or pathological attitudes and it is this aspect which is the concern of the psychoanalyst. When the degree of expression of anger, rage, hate, or hostility is out of all proportion to the appar-ent immediate inciting cause, we are dealing with something

which goes beyond immediate self-preservation; in fact, it is often self-destructive. However, even irrational behavior usually has an understandable beginning. Just as normal hostility has its origin in justifiable fear of real danger, irrational hostility has its origin in anxiety. As Horney has pointed out, anxiety is often coped with by hostility, but the hostility, by creating difficulties in relationships, produces new anxiety, so that there is an ever-increasing burden of anxiety and hostility.

(p. 11)

What if she would have seen systemic oppression as the "concern of the psychoanalyst"? That may have led to her activism. Thompson's activism was invested in the belief that science would lead the way to a better society—something she very much wanted. We might call her an optimist, while those around her at the time thought of her as a pragmatist. She acknowledges the inequality and hostility shown to people of color in the United States and the justifiable anger that comes with that mistreatment, but the complexity is hard to hold on to as she tries to think analytically, seeming to ask, what can the psychoanalyst offer?

In another essay, "An Introduction to Minor Maladjustments" (1959), she again enters into an uncommon clinical discussion of race relations, naming what she sees as a cultural "hazard" present in society—one addressed by Fromm in *The Sane Society* (1955). Here, Thompson again offers a clinical example to explain what she identifies as a social-psychological trap. She writes:

If one has subscribed to the importance of being successful, being what is expected of him with the hope of winning power, it is very disrupting to personal integrity and even to sanity if the price of this means denial of valued basic principles. An example is the following: a man, believing in the rights of Negros, is in a position of authority in a Southern state. He can belligerently espouse the cause of Negros and probably, thereby, lose whatever status he has. He thinks maybe he should take a middle-of-the-road course—but then he becomes confused. Is he deciding upon his course because it will produce the best results in the long run, or is he influenced by his personal ambition to be accepted and win a more impressive position in the community? The state of conflict between the two ideas develops, so that he no longer is able to decide what is best for the cause of the Negros, the cause to which he thought he was dedicated. What got in the way was his marketing need for personal success, and his final choice was determined by his personal ambition. But some part of him could not accept his decision, and presently he consulted a psychiatrist because of depression and suicidal thoughts. In stating his problem, he said "I cannot understand why I am so unhappy. So far, I have accomplished everything I set out to do, and it looks as if I would get the next position I am seeking." Because he was a person unusually honest with himself, the cause of his unhappiness soon was made clear to him. The issue here is not whether the more effective course is to be radical or middle of the road, but the fact that the need to be successful personally was obscuring his judgment. This man might have gone on to the end of his days, pursuing his personal ambitions without realizing their marketing character, if he had not come into conflict with the prejudices of his community, which forced him to face his values.

(Thompson, 1959, pp. 197–198)

Fromm's influence is apparent in Thompson's analysis, specifically in her use of the term "marketing character," but the courage to pursue the topic of race in clinical psychoanalysis is purely Thompson. Her unique use of Fromm's terminology speaks to the deep cross-fertilization of ideas between Thompson, Sullivan, Horney, and Fromm. Thompson makes clear she is talking about people who suffer from compromises they have made in order to *adapt*, not people who *fail* to *adapt*, an important distinction in psychiatry. She suggests that both types suffer from their need for approval. Conforming with authority to received approval and acceptance promotes, in this case, a public racist attitude.

Twentieth Century Liberalism: Successes and Failures

Thompson and her colleagues were a small group of liberals in a sea of conservatives. Naoko Wake (2011) points to how their attempts at promoting their liberal attitudes fell short of their aspirations. In fact, their unconscious attitudes, Wake argues, added to the rise of conservatism in the United States. Despite turning away from the 19th century codification of people as immature, pathological, and diseased toward a more-alike-than-different attitude publicly, for some, their private, mostly unconscious attitudes remained unexamined. Wake contends that in many cases, they were sexual minorities themselves with anti-homosexual or racist attitudes. Unexamined internalized homophobia and racism hampered their cause. In some cases, their private attitudes were liberal while their public personas were conservative. Wake suggests an interesting hypothesis—that this gap prevented mainstream public activism and shored up homophobic and racist policies.

Prejudice and bias have a deep history in American life. They stand in contrast to the aspiration of a country as a beacon of liberty and justice for all—as the Puritans preached. Rather, the United States is a country where slavery, gender inequality, xenophobia, and anti-homosexual attitudes flourished unabated—as they still do in many ways. Thompson and her closest friends were entangled in and enacted these cultural conflicts. For example, Thompson's friend, the anthropologist Ruth Benedict, was trapped in a public and private dissonance. On the one hand, Benedict focused on the "bias against homosexuality as socially constructed bigotry" (Wake, 2011, p. 130). She argued in "Anthropology and the Abnormal" (1934) that the stigmatization of homosexuality must be changed:

> A tendency toward [homosexuality] in our culture exposes an individual to all the conflicts...and we tend to identify the consequences of this conflict with homosexuality. But these consequences are obviously local and cultural...Whenever homosexuality has been given an honorable place in any society, those to whom it is congenial have filled adequately the honorable roles.
>
> (p. 64)

However, privately, Benedict sought to keep her relationship with Margaret Mead secret, much the way that Sullivan kept his gay partnership with James (Jimmie) Inscoe mostly secret. Since homosexuality was illegal, they had little choice but to remain silent. That silence had unintended consequences.

There is a deeply layered complexity and tension contained in these examples. One that is relevant to Thompson's private life revolves around her housekeeper, Lillie Fisher, an African American woman who spent much of her life in Thompson's employ. Thompson had a deep emotional attachment to Lillie. After Lillie retired, she revealed in a letter to Erich Fromm dated March 11, 1965 (housed in the Erich Fromm Archive, Tuebingen), that for the first time in many years she felt "alone in the big world. No mother." From Thompson's perspective, Lillie had devoted her life to taking care of her and Lillie had no one else in the world: "I am all she has," she tells Fromm.[11] When Thompson died, she left an account in the State Mutual Building Association of Baltimore to Lillie Fisher—a sign of her love, gratitude, and respect. In the will, Fisher is identified only as her "maid."

In many respects, Lillie and Clara were intimate equals who respected each other in defiance of conventional norms. On the other hand, one cannot ignore the resonance in the term "maid" as the well-known connection to the "house slave"—apparent in the numerous critiques of *The Help*—and that aspects of these were perhaps unknowingly replicated on Clara's part, and perhaps not unknowingly on the part of Lillie, who most likely would not feel free to bring up these feelings. And yet Fisher was seen as a nurturing maternal figure who took care of Thompson's household and looked after her as well. Thompson's colleague Silverberg (1959) memorably recalled Fisher's "southern cooking and her utter loyalty to Thompson. Her loyalty sometimes took the form of petulant scolding, which Clara bore with great equanimity. Her relationship with Lilly [sp] endured throughout nearly her entire life" (p. 3).

Who was Lillie Fisher? Fisher was born in 1882. She was ten years older than Thompson. She was close to her own sister, Lottie Taylor, who lived in Baltimore. The 1930 US Census lists Lillie Fisher as a widow who married at age 28. She had no schooling and was a cook. She is listed as living with her sister and her husband. She would have been in her late 30s when she went to work for Thompson in the 1920s. According to Thompson's will, Fisher was living in Baltimore when Thompson died. The address listed is a townhouse in one of Baltimore's earliest African American middle-class neighborhoods. Fisher returned to her community following her retirement. What does that tell us about her connection to Thompson?

Thompson benefited from her relationship with Fisher, and Fisher stayed in her employment, but how did they perceive their differences? Could their relationship have been devoid of racism? Thompson cared for—indeed possibly loved—Lillie (or at least loved her carefully constructed image of Lillie, an image that Lillie had to help maintain and play into), a sentiment inferred in her letter to Fromm, but did she know her? Did she know how connected Lillie was to her family? When Lillie died, her sister wrote that she was surrounded by friends and family. Her obituary paints a different picture than the one Thompson suggests: "my heart ached more for her than for me," and "why do parents have to be so hurt?" Lillie was returning to an extended network that appears to have been loving and supportive. The relationship between Thompson and Fisher holds much complexity and a fair amount of "not-knowing."

Thompson also boldly took up the messy construct and cultural attitudes toward homosexuality. Her essay "Changing Concepts of Homosexuality in Psychoanalysis" (1947) presents groundbreaking ideas that run in two different directions.

> The different cultural attitudes toward the sissy and the tomboy again show society's greater tolerance for the female homosexual type. When a boy is called a Sissy, he feels stigmatized, and the group considers that it has been belittled him. No such disapproval goes with a girl's being called a tomboy. In fact, she often feels considerable pride in the fact. Probably the names get their value from childhood ideas that courage and daring are desirable traits in both sexes. So, the sissy is a coward, a mama's boy, and the tomboy, is a brave girl who can hold her own with a boy her size. These attitudes probably became a part of later attitudes toward homosexuality in the two sexes.
>
> (p. 186)

She declares, "various personality problems may find partial solution in a homosexual symptom, but nothing has been shown as specifically producing homosexuality" (p. 188).

We can hear the reverberations of her friendships with Sullivan and Benedict reflected in her statement:

People who for reasons external to their own personality find their choice of love object limited to their own sex may be said to be "normal homosexuals," in the sense that they utilized the best type of interpersonal relationship available to them. These people are not the problem of psychopathology.

(p. 186)

To their credit, Thompson like Benedict, and Sullivan, struggled to confront sexism and racism despite the limitations of their era. They were bolstered perhaps by their personal values and by the social sciences.

Returning to the social sciences, Thompson (1950c) argued the American psychiatrists that went to Europe brought something new to American Psychoanalysis. They had already been trained in the importance of the environment as a contribution to mental illness, so they interpreted Freud's system less literally than the Europeans. She writes:

About 1930 a few analysts had begun to show a new kind of interest in anthropological studies of culture, and one anthropologist, Edward Sapir, was a pioneer in advocating collaboration of anthropology, sociology and psychoanalysis.

(p. 194)

The Relevance of Thompson's Work

Thompson was a pioneer who broke many boundaries and delivered a new psychoanalysis to American shores. She advocated for a therapeutic method that was more equal and highlighted the mutually influencing character of the work. She was willing to take on controversial topics such as race, gender, and sexuality. While the conforming nature of her early family experience were felt restrictions that she needed to escape, the ideas about equality and fairness endured. They became her true north, driving her opinions about equality, mutuality, and fairness. Her 1938 essay extolling the psychoanalytic significance of the choice of analyst set the stage for how the analyst's personality is critical in the analytic process. Over time, her clinical concepts became a pillar of psychoanalytic work, though she does not receive due credit. Echoes of Thompson's work are heard in her analysand, Benjamin Wolstein, who in his interview with Irwin Hirsch (2000) acknowledges that he learned from her the concept of "direct experience." Levenson's work (see 1992) also reverberates with Thompson's themes, specifically the role of the total personality of the analyst and the necessity of trust in the analytic encounter (1938). Perhaps she would strongly agree with Stern (1996), who maintains that beliefs are values; they assert what is important in life, and in psychoanalytic treatment, they become the engine that makes things happen. Thompson's values drove her to seek changes in herself and in her patients. Her ideas are the forerunner for what we have come to understand as therapeutic action. Not only did she make significant contributions to the clinical literature, she was also an organizational leader at a time when psychoanalytic politics included many wars with various schisms, all of which she navigated with class. Thompson was the first director of The William Alanson White Institute of Psychiatry, as it was called in 1946, and served through the years when it received a permanent charter as The William Alanson White Institute of Psychiatry, Psychoanalysis and Psychology in 1951. She was at the helm until her death in 1958 at the young age of 65.

Notes

1. An American brand of psychoanalysis is reported to be more optimistic and more moralistic than the continental view that is closer to Freud's. See Hale, 1995, p. 379.
2. Pembroke was the women's college of Brown University.
3. Thompson's analysis with Ferenczi occurred over the summers of 1928 for two months, 1929 for two months, and 1930 for three months; she then moved to Budapest from 1931 to 1933.
4. Paper originally presented on March 15, 1955 for the Harry Stack Sullivan Society.
5. I take up this complex and complicated issue in *Clara Thompson: The Life and Work of an American Psychoanalyst (1893–1933)* (in press).
6. This paper, first titled "What is Penis Envy?" was presented at the first annual convention of the Association for the Advancement of Psychoanalysis in Boston, May 19, 1942.

7. *The Role of Women in This Culture* (1941) was Thompson's first paper on the psychology of women.
8. The patient in this vignette may have been Maurice Green; how else could he have been able to report the event verbatim?
9. It is worth noting that Joseph "Snake" Thompson was a man of considerable talents. He had a depth of knowledge in a variety of fields, from Asian religion to zoology. He was known as "Snake" because of his interest in herpetology, and he was a founder of the San Diego Zoo. He was also a recognized breeder of Siamese cats and was instrumental in developing the Burmese breed.
10. Thompson resigned from Adolf Meyer's clinic. He accused her taking patients from the clinic into her practice. Clara Thompson also found her first treatment to be of little use, and she followed it with what she called an almost 100 percent positive analysis with Ferenczi.
11. This letter, dated March 11, 1956, is housed at the Erich Fromm Archive in Tuebingen, Germany and these excerpts are printed here by permission of Rainer Funk, Director of the Archive.

References

Benedict, R. (1934). Anthropology and the abnormal. *Journal of General Psychology, 10*(1), 59–82.

Benedict, R. (1938). Continuities and discontinuities in cultural conditioning. *Psychiatry, 1*(2), 161–167.

Capelle, E. L. (1993). Analyzing the "modern woman": Psychoanalytic debates about feminism, 1920–1950 [Unpublished doctoral dissertation]. Columbia University.

Conci, M. (2012). *Sullivan revisited – Life and work: Harry Stack Sullivan's relevance for contemporary psychiatry, psychotherapy and psychoanalysis.* Trento: Tangram Ediz Scientifiche.

Cushing, F. H. (1922 [1998]). *My adventures in Zuni.* Trento, Italy, USA: Filter Press.

D'Ercole, A. (2017). The repossession of the interpersonal tradition: On holding close our transdisciplinary roots. *Contemporary Psychoanalysis, 53*(1), 95–111.

D'Ercole, A. (in press). *Clara Thompson: The life and work of an American psychoanalyst.* New York: Routledge Press.

Dooley, L. (1938). The genesis of psychological sex differences. *Psychiatry, 1*(2), 181–195.

Dupont, J. (Ed.) (1988). *The clinical diary of Sándor Ferenczi* (M. Balint & N. Z. Jackson, Trans.). Cambridge: Harvard University Press. (Originally published in 1932)

Eissler, K., & Thompson, C. (1952). Interviews and recollections, Set A, 1914–1998 with K. R. Eissler/Interviewer, Sigmund Freud Papers (Box 115). Washington, DC: Manuscripts Division, Library of Congress.

Eliot, G. (1860). *Mill on the floss*. London: William Blackwood and Sons.

Ferenczi, S. (1928). The elasticity of the psychoanalytic technique. In S. Ferenczi, *Final contributions to the problems and methods of psycho-analysis* (pp. 87–101). London: Karnac Books.

Friedman, L. J. (2013). *The lives of Erich Fromm: Love's Prophet*. New York: Columbia University Press.

Fromm, E. (1955). *The sane society*. New York: Rinehart & Company Inc.

Frosch, J. (1991). The New York psychoanalytic civil wars. *Journal of the American Psychoanalytic Association, 39*, 1037–1064.

Gabbard, G. O. (2016). *Boundaries and boundary violations in psychoanalysis*. Washington, DC: American Psychiatric Publications.

Green, M.R. (Ed.) (1964). *Interpersonal psychoanalysis: The selected papers of Clara M. Thompson*. New York: Basic Books.

Hale, N. (1995). *The rise and crisis of psychoanalysis in the United States: Freud and the Americans 1917–1985*. New York: Oxford University Press.

Hirsch, I. (2000). Interview with Benjamin Wolstein. *Contemporary Psychoanalysis, 36*, 187–232.

Horney, K. (1939). *New ways in psychoanalysis*. New York: W.W. Norton & Co.

Levenson, E. A. (1992). Harry Stack Sullivan: From interpersonal psychiatry to interpersonal psychoanalysis. *Contemporary Psychoanalysis, 28*, 450–466.

Levenson, E. A. (2009). The enigma of the transference. *Contemporary Psychoanalysis, 45*(2), 163–178.

Malinowski, B. (1922 [2013]). *Argonauts of the western Pacific*. Long Grove, Illinois: Waveland Press.

Menaker, E. (1989). *Appointment in Vienna*. New York: St. Martin's Press.

Perry, H. S. (1982). *Psychiatrist of America: The life of Harry Stack Sullivan*. Boston: Belknap Press.

Peters, M. (1979). Biographies of women. *Biography, 2*(3), 201–217.

Rachman, A. W. (1997). *Sándor Ferenczi: The psychotherapist of tenderness and passion*. New York: Jason Aronson.

Rachman, A. W. (2018). *Elizabeth Severn: The "evil" genius of psychoanalysis*. Oxon, Ox: Routledge.

Rudnytsky, P. L. (2015). The other side of the story: Severn on Ferenczi and mutual analysis. In A. Harris & S. Kuchuck (Eds.), *The legacy of Sandor Ferenczi: From ghost to ancestor* (pp. 134–149). London: Routledge.

Shapiro, S. A. (1993). Clara Thompson: Ferenczi's messenger with half a message. In L. Aron & A. Harris (Eds.), *The legacy of Sandor Ferenczi* (pp. 159–174). Hillsdale, NJ: The Analytic Press.

Silverberg, W. V. (1959). Clara Thompson memorial. *The Newsletter of the White Institute, 7*(1), 1.

Stern, D. B. (1996). The social construction of therapeutic action. *Psychoanalytic Inquiry, 16*(2), 265–293.

Thompson, C. (1938). Notes on the psychoanalytic significance of the choice of analyst. *Psychiatry: Journal of the Biology and the Pathology of Interpersonal Relations, 1,* 205–216.

Thompson, C. (1941). The role of women in this culture. *Psychiatry: Journal of the Biology and the Pathology of Interpersonal Relations, 4,* 1–8.

Thompson, C. (1942). Cultural pressures in the psychology of women. *Psychiatry: Journal of the Biology and the Pathology of Interpersonal Relations, 5,* 331–339.

Thompson, C. (1943b). "Penis envy" in women. *Psychiatry: Journal of the Biology and the Pathology of Interpersonal Relations, 6,* 123–125.

Thompson, C. (1943a). 'The therapeutic technique of Sándor Ferenczi:' A comment. *International Journal of Psychoanalysis, 24,* 64–66.

Thompson, C. (1947). Changing concepts of homosexuality in psychoanalysis. *Psychiatry: Journal of the Biology and the Pathology of Interpersonal Relations, 10,* 183–189.

Thompson, C. (1950a). Some effects of the derogatory attitude towards female sexuality. *Psychiatry, 13*(3), 349–354.

Thompson, C. (1950b). Cultural complications in the sexual life of woman. In *Feminine psychology: Its implications for psychoanalytic medicine.* Symposium Proceedings, March 18 (Vol. 19).

Thompson, C. (1950c). *Psychoanalysis: Evolution and development.* New York: Hermitage.

Thompson, C. (1956, March 11). Letter to Erich Fromm. Housed in the Erich Fromm Archive, Courtesy of Rainer Funk, Erich Fromm Archive, Tuebingen.

Thompson, C. (1959). An introduction to minor maladjustments. In S. Arieti (Ed.), *American handbook of psychiatry* (pp. 237–244). New York: Basic Books.

Thompson, C. (1964). The interpersonal approach to the clinical problems of masochism. In M.R. Green (Ed.), *Interpersonal psychoanalysis: The selected papers of Clara M. Thompson* (pp. 183–198). New York: Basic Books.

Thompson, C. (1988). Sándor Ferenczi, 1873–1933. *Contemporary Psychoanalysis, 24*(2), 182–195.

Thompson, C. (2017). The history of the William Alanson White Institute. *Contemporary Psychoanalysis*, *53*, 1–6.

Wake, N. (2011). *Private practices: Harry Stack Sullivan, the science of homosexuality, and American liberalism*. New Brunswick, NJ: Rutgers University Press.

Waugaman, R. M. (2016). Further notes on choosing an analyst. *Psychiatry*, *79*(1), 13–18.

Weiss, F. A., Zuger, B., Thompson, C., Landman, L., & Meerloo, J. A. M. (1959). Dynamics of hostility: A panel discussion. *American Journal of Psychoanalysis*, *19*(1), 4–27.

Chapter 9

Psychoanalysis in the Shadow of Fascism and Genocide

Erich Fromm and the Interpersonal Tradition

Roger Frie

In 1939, shortly before the start of World War II, Karl Menninger wrote a heated letter to the editor of the new journal *Psychiatry*. Menninger was a leading member of Freudian establishment and strongly objected to a recent article by Erich Fromm, arguing that it "misrepresented Freud" and contained "egregious errors." He went on to say that Fromm's article was causing "a great many uncomplimentary things" to be said about the journal's "misrepresentation of psychoanalysis" and that it should not stand "unrefuted" (cited in Perry, 1982, p. 381). Sullivan came to Fromm's defence, responding firmly but politely, "I am much distressed by your reaction to Dr. Fromm's article," adding that "Dr. Fromm's merits" are not in question. The aim of *Psychiatry*, Sullivan concluded, is "to represent the best" (cited in Perry, 1982, p. 382).

The letter exchange between Menninger and Sullivan was part of a larger struggle for psychoanalytic supremacy that would isolate interpersonal psychoanalysis from the mainstream for decades to come. It also points to the centrality of Fromm's contributions and to Sullivan's strong support of his friend and colleague. Given Fromm's fame as a mid-century public intellectual and social critic, it is easy to overlook his role as a pioneering psychoanalyst. In fact, Fromm's psychoanalytic practice was perhaps the one constant in life that spanned different disciplines, continents, cultures and languages. Over the course of his long career, Fromm (1900–1980) co-founded psychoanalytic institutes and organizations including the South German Institute for Psychoanalysis in Frankfurt in 1929, the William Alanson White

DOI: 10.4324/9781003270355-10

Institute in New York in 1943 and the International Federation of Psychoanalytic Societies in 1962.[1]

The chapter begins by tracing the development of Fromm's psychoanalytic writings in Germany and the United States during the decade of the 1930s. In contrast to most of his psychoanalytic colleagues, Fromm's dual training as a sociologist and psychoanalyst prepared him to comment on the social and political crises of the day. Fromm's sociopsychological approach formed the basis for his timely and trenchant account of the "authoritarian character" in *Escape from Freedom* (1941). Then I return to Fromm's 1939 controversial article and examine his relationship with Sullivan. Fromm and Sullivan were connected by their shared passion for interdisciplinary scholarship and by their belief in the necessity of taking a stand on vital political issues. I examine Fromm's public opposition to fascism and Sullivan's stance against anti-Semitism and link them to the tragic private history of Fromm's family members in Nazi Germany that was unfolding simultaneously. Above all, I suggest that Fromm's life and work serve as an important reminder that interpersonal psychoanalysis emerged out of a period of social and geopolitical turmoil and that this beginning also makes it uniquely suited to respond to the crises we face today. With this in mind, I conclude by discussing the contemporary resonance of Fromm's examination of racial narcissism and the development of a socially engaged psychoanalysis.

Psychoanalysis and Social Character

The trajectory of Fromm's life (1900–1980) was shaped by the traumas and tragedies of the twentieth century. Fromm was born in and grew up in the city of Frankfurt in an orthodox German Jewish family.[2] He was the only child of Nephtali, a wine merchant, and Rosa (née Krause) Fromm. At an early age, Fromm demonstrated an interest in the study of the Talmud and drew inspiration from his rabbinic ancestors. On his father's side, his great-grandfather (Selig Bär Bamberger) was one of the most prominent and learned German rabbis of the mid-nineteenth century, and his grandfather (Rabbi Seligmann Pinchas Fromm) was a leader of the Frankfurt Jewish community. His mother had an uncle (Ludwig Krause) who was likewise a well-known Talmudist and became Fromm's first Talmudic teacher.

As a young man, Fromm was alarmed by the nationalist fervor that gripped Germany during the First World War. He found solace and inspiration in Jewish thinking and learning and joined a growing circle around Rabbi Nehemiah Nobel that included the young philosopher Franz Rosenzweig and such eminent figures as Martin Buber and Gershom Scholem. In 1918, Fromm began studying law at the University of Frankfurt but soon switched to sociology and transferred to the University of Heidelberg. He received his doctorate in sociology in 1922, where he was supervised by the well-known sociologist, Alfred Weber (the brother of Max Weber); he was taught psychology by Karl Jaspers and philosophy by Heinz Rickert.

In addition to religion and sociology, Fromm became interested in psychoanalysis. When Fromm was in Heidelberg, he entered a psychoanalytic treatment with Frieda Reichmann, but it ended after they fell in love. Fromm and Reichman married in 1926, well before the establishment of the kind of ethical norms that govern psychoanalytic practice today. Together they founded a psychoanalytically oriented sanatorium in Heidelberg (*das Therapeutikum*), gave up their Jewish orthodoxy and developed a secular and humanistic outlook.[3] Reichmann supported Fromm when he underwent an analysis with Wilhelm Wittenberg in Munich, which was subsequently followed by a period of supervision with Karl Landauer at the Southwest German Psychoanalytic Study Group in Frankfurt. In order to finish his psychoanalytic training, Fromm moved to Berlin in 1928, where he completed a training analysis with Hanns Sachs, a personal friend of Freud's and one of the earliest psychoanalysts.

During the 1920s, Berlin had become the European center for innovative arts and culture. This was Berlin before the onset of the Nazis, before Goebbels and his Brownshirts could impose their racist ideology at will. The city embraced a culture of permissiveness and experimentation and exemplified the liberal and democratic outlook of Weimar Germany. Psychoanalysis thrived there. The Berlin Psychoanalytic Institute was at the forefront of the psychoanalytic movement. Among its faculty and candidates were such luminaries as Abraham, Alexander, Fenichel, Groddeck, Horney, Jacobson, Klein, Rado, Sachs and Spitz. The Freudian technique used by many of these analysts would have been familiar to American mainstream psychoanalysts in the post-war decades. But their left-wing politics and commitment to working with lower socioeconomic classes probably would not.

Fromm's academic background in sociology enabled him to comment on the events around him. In 1928, he presented a paper on "Psychoanalysis of the Petty Bourgeoisie," a topic that would soon find expression in his research on the authoritarian tendencies of German workers. In 1929, Fromm gave a lecture in Frankfurt on "Psychoanalysis and Sociology" (see Fromm, 1930), which was a preliminary attempt to create a synthesis between Freud and Marx. This essay demonstrates a key theme in his work, namely understanding and explaining the process of socialization. His work brought him to the attention of Max Horkheimer, the director the Institute for Social Research (later known as the Frankfurt School), who invited him to join. Horkheimer recognized Fromm's psychoanalytic prowess, and under the auspices of the Institute, Fromm began his project of integrating Marxism and psychoanalysis.

By 1930, Fromm had been certified by the German Psychoanalytic Society (DPG) and he set off on a career of combining social analysis with psychoanalytic practice. The increasingly turbulent political events in Germany at the time influenced the trajectory of his work and life. It was in response to the rise of fascism that Fromm embarked on one of his most important early works: a study of the character structure of the German working class during the late Weimar Republic. Fromm and his institute associates handed out 3,300 lengthy questionnaires in Berlin and Frankfurt to workers who were identified as socialist. While only 1,100 responses were collected, the results suggested that only a small percentage (15%) of the respondents demonstrated clear anti-authoritarian beliefs. In other words, workers who were presumed to be solidly against authoritarianism revealed pro-fascist tendencies. Fromm's first book, *Escape from Freedom*, would seek to understand the appeal of authoritarianism and provide a means to understand the collapse of German workers' parties during the rise of Nazism. But as it turned out, the results of the workers' study did not mesh with the Institute's Marxist outlook, nor did Horkheimer believe it to be sufficiently representative of the Institute's perspectives (on both points, see McLaughlin, 1999, 2017). It was shelved and remained unpublished until the 1980s (see Fromm, 1984), despite forming the largely unacknowledged basis for Theodore Adorno's well-known post-war study, *The Authoritarian Personality* (1950).

Throughout the 1930s, Fromm's research sought to show how people are shaped by socioeconomic class, religion and ideology. According to Fromm, societies are structured in such a way that individuals take on the roles their particular society requires of them. He was particularly interested in demonstrating how society produces persons who unconsciously adapt to meet society's economic needs even though these may conflict with our own emotional well-being. As Fromm would famously remark in a later work: "It is the function of social character to shape the energies of the members of society in such a way that their behavior is not left to conscious decisions whether or not to follow the social pattern but that *people want to act as they have to act*" (Fromm, 1949, p. 5, original emphasis).

In the process of laying out his sociopsychological approach, Fromm became increasingly critical of Freudian psychoanalysis. In his 1934 article, *The Theory of Mother Right and its Relevance for Social Psychology*, Fromm questioned the centrality of the Oedipus complex, and the primacy of the patriarchal social structure in

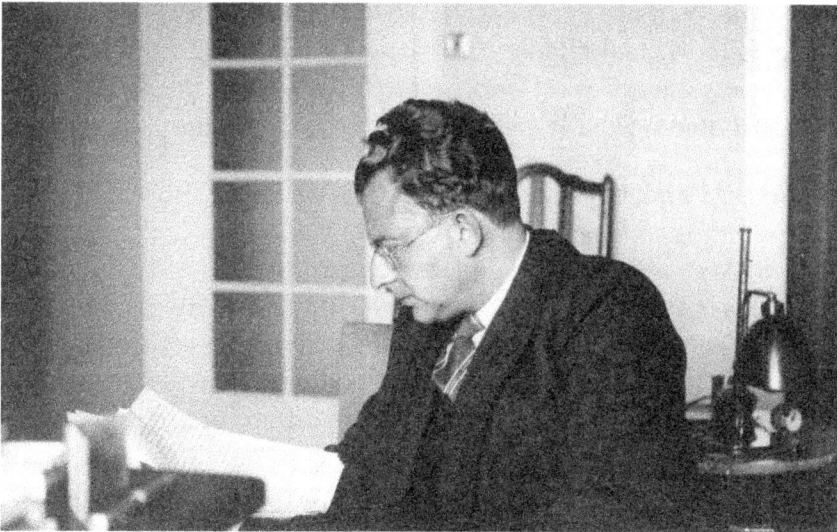

Figure 9 Erich Fromm in a rare photograph from the 1930s, ©Literary Estate of Erich Fromm, Tübingen.

Freud's work. In place of libidinal stages of development, Fromm began to conceive of human development in terms of imagined and actual relations with other people. In 1936, he wrote to his colleague Karl August Wittfogel, "Those urges which motivate social activities are not, as Freud supposes, sublimations of sexual instincts, but rather products of social processes. These urges ... are not to be understood biologically, but rather as in the context of the practice of social living ... Freud has wrongly based psychology totally on natural factors" (cited in Funk, 2019, p. 53).

This line of questioning finds its fullest expression in Fromm's article, *Man's Impulse Structure and its Relation to Culture* (1937). Fromm focuses above all on the limitations that follow from Freud's emphasis on the drives. He takes issue with Freud's biologically determined account of human nature which is unable to account for the social and cultural factors in the shaping of the person. For example, Fromm solidly rejects Freud's psychology of women, which he argues is effectively a means of rationalizing patriarchy. He suggests that the patriarchal family is itself a product of specific social constellation in society and becomes the means by which the child is socialized into the values of that of society. Fromm's perspective was informed by Karen Horney's writings on feminine psychology at the time as well as his own observations of mid-1930s European and American white, heterosexual middle-class society.[4] The point, for Fromm, is that society was always at work in the person, so that the person exists only as a fundamentally social being. As Fromm states:

> Society and the individual are not "opposite" to each other. *Society is nothing but living, concrete individuals, and the individual exists only as a social human being.* His individual life practice is necessarily determined by the life practice of his society or class and, in the last analysis, by the manner of production of his society, that is, how this society produces, how it is organized to satisfy the needs of its members. The differences in the manner of production and life of various societies or classes lead to the development of different character structures typical of the particular society. Various societies differ from each other not only in differences in manner of production and social and political

organization but also in that their people exhibit a typical character structure despite all individual differences. We shall call this
"the socially typical character."

(Fromm, [1937] 2010, p. 58, original italics)

Fromm thus positions the person within social, cultural and political
relations in order to reveal the effect that these forces can have. By
virtue of our participation in society, we learn to contain thoughts
and feelings that might otherwise challenge the status quo. In this
way, we might say that society inscribes pathology into human relationships. For Fromm, the goal of psychoanalysis was not simply to
adapt to society's needs, but to embrace a more grounded and ethi-
cally centered stance, in essence, to live soundly against the stream.

Not surprisingly, Fromm's critical viewpoint found little sympathy among his Freudian colleagues. When Fromm submitted *Man's
Impulse Structure and its Relation to Culture* for publication to the
journal of the Institute for Social Research, it was soundly rejected.
Fromm's evolving understanding of psychoanalysis clashed with the
increasingly orthodox Freudian position represented by the Institute.
Fromm and Horkheimer had long enjoyed a cordial relationship and
Fromm played a key part in helping the Institute move from their
temporary exile in Geneva to a more permanent home at Columbia
University. But growing differences in their interpretations of Marx
and Freud, made worse by Fromm's acrimonious interactions with
Theodore Adorno, meant that there was little future for him at the
Institute. As a result, after 1939, Fromm was largely written out of
the history of the Frankfurt School (Institute for Social Research),
despite his formative early role (see McLaughlin, 1999, 2017).

The further Fromm ventured from Freud, the closer his associations with other like-minded psychoanalysts became. Fromm first
met Sullivan in 1934, soon after arriving in the United States. Their
relationship blossomed as each discovered how much he could learn
from the other. Sullivan became acquainted with Fromm's empirical
study on German workers, his sociopsychological perspective and his
critique of Freudian psychoanalysis. Fromm, in turn, learned about
the ways in which Sullivan conceptualized the self in a nexus of interpersonal relations and was introduced to the culture and personality

movement. As Clara Thompson later remarked in her 1956 article *Sullivan and Fromm*, "The work of each supplements the other, and their basic assumptions about human beings are similar. The chief area which they share in common is the interest in the impact of cultural pressures on personality development. The chief area of difference is in theories about the self" (Thompson [1956] 1979, p. 195).

In 1937, when the American Psychoanalytic Association began to require its members to be medical doctors, Sullivan sought to assure Fromm of a psychoanalytic life outside of the mainstream and invited Fromm to teach in the newly established Washington School of Psychiatry, which he gladly accepted. Fromm's psychoanalytic associations in New York consisted of friends and colleagues, new and old, including Sullivan, Horney, Thompson, Fromm-Reichman and others, who met on a weekly basis and formed the so-called Zodiac group. It was through Sullivan that Fromm also met and interacted with like-minded interdisciplinary researchers. Among this number were the anthropologists Ruth Benedict, Abram Kardiner, Margaret Mead and Edward Sapir, along with a host of social scientists (see Wake 2011 and Wake, this volume). The influence of anthropology on Fromm, Sullivan and Horney led their combined work to become known as "cultural psychoanalysis," a label that would hold long after the split between Fromm and Horney in 1941 and the founding of the W.A. White Institute in 1943 (see Frie, 2014).

Thus, in 1939, when Fromm's article *The Social Philosophy of 'Will Therapy'* appeared in *Psychiatry*, Fromm and Sullivan had already been working closely together for five years. The fact that Sullivan published the article despite the opposition it would surely face speaks to the importance he placed on it. Sullivan's subsequent defense of Fromm points to the high esteem in which he held his colleague. Given Menninger's complaint, it is easy to assume that Fromm's article was a lengthy and critical exegesis of Freud's texts. In fact, Fromm's account of Freud forms only a small part of the discussion, the chief purpose of which is to examine the work of Otto Rank. But it is what Fromm says about Freud in those few brief pages that matters (the following quotes from Fromm's 1939 article are from pp. 230–232).

Fromm's stated aim is to analyze Freud's social philosophy in order "to illustrate the general point that a psychological system is rooted in certain philosophical premises." His critical discussion of Freud articulates many of the points for which interpersonal psychoanalysis has since become known. Fromm covers a range of topics, but in the main, his arguments are aimed at Freud's neglect of the interpersonal dimension. According to Fromm, Freud's focus on the drives and on early childhood experience is achieved at the expense of accounting for the wider social "milieu." As Fromm states, Freud's "instinctivistic approach" is in "some contradiction" with the social surround. In this sense, Fromm continues, Freudian psychoanalysis is "not consistent with the progressive, philosophical premise of environmental determination." Fromm also expresses concern about the degree to which Freudian psychoanalysis ends up helping the individual to simply adapt to the needs of society. As Fromm writes, the "ability to play the role in society which the individual is supposed to play, to be able to function smoothly as a cog in a big machine, is essentially what [Freud's] 'capacity for work' implies." In other words, Fromm is concerned that psychoanalysis may end up serving the needs of a society that inscribes pathology into human relationships. Fromm's critique also extends to psychoanalytic technique, particularly the notion of neutrality, which Fromm likens to the attitude of medical doctor who looks at the patient as though he or she were an object for study and examination. The problem, according to Fromm, is that "one cannot help anyone emotionally... if one remains distant and looks at him [or her] as an object." As Fromm concludes, "There is no psychological understanding if we do not make a move, if we do not reach out toward the person whom we want to understand."[5]

Escape from Freedom

Two years later, Fromm published his first major work, *Escape from Freedom*. Fromm includes an Appendix entitled, "Character and Social Process," in which he elaborates his psychoanalytic position contra Freud and explicitly allies himself with Sullivan. As Fromm states,

> The fundamental approach to human personality is the understanding of the human being's relationship to the world, to others, to nature, and to him or herself. We believe that the human being is primarily a social being, and not, as Freud assumes, primarily self-sufficient and only secondarily in need of others in order to

satisfy his or her instinctual needs. *In this sense, we believe that individual psychology is fundamentally social psychology, or in Sullivan's terms, the psychology of interpersonal relationships.*
(Fromm, 1941, p. 290, my emphasis)

This is perhaps the best articulation to date of the emerging interpersonal position that unites Fromm and Sullivan. Fromm's express aim is to show how the social character of a group "determines the thinking, feeling and acting of individuals who belong to that group." This is essentially the inverse of any psychology that takes as its staring point the individual person and only secondarily accounts for the existence of social factors.

Fromm's approach in *Escape from Freedom* demonstrates his clear proximity to Sullivan, but it also reveals the presence of Horney's ideas. For example, Fromm's analysis of the causes of authoritarianism is anticipated by Horney in her 1939 article, *Can You Take a Stand?* Horney suggests that the conditions needed for fascism to thrive may stem a sense of self-alienation and a shifting of "the center of gravity from self to others" that actually begins in childhood. According to Horney, "this state of mind has important social implications, for it makes people 'enormously susceptible' to totalitarianism" (Horney, 1939, cited in Paris, 2000, p. 225). In an evocative passage, Horney analyzes the allure fascism:

> Fascist ideology promises to fulfill all their needs. The individual in a fascist state is not supposed to stand up for his own wishes, rights, judgments. Decisions and judgments of value are made for him and he has merely to follow. He can forget about his own weakness by adoring the leader. His ego is bolstered up by being submerged in the greater unity of race and nation
> (Horney, 1939, cited in Paris, 2000, p. 226)

Escape from Freedom was published in 1941, just as the United States officially declared war on Germany and Japan. The book met with great success and spoke to an American readership that was eager for an explanation that of Germany's enthusiastic embrace of Hitler. Fromm employed a broad historical narrative to draw a stark contrast between democracy and totalitarian regimes. He argued that modern European society had ushered in new freedoms and laid the conditions for the emergence of the autonomous and rationale individuals. But with these changes came a deep-rooted anxiety and a feeling of isolation. People were faced with a choice: to engage productively with other human beings and garner the benefits of society (democracy) or escape a sense of fear and loneliness by submitting to a greater authority (totalitarianism).

The German experience of defeat in the First World War and the economic and societal crises in the years that followed had created deep-seated anxiety, thus setting the stage for Hitler and the Nazi party. According to Fromm, the rise of authoritarian thinking in Germany during the 1930s was characterized by the simultaneous presence of sadism and masochism. "Sadism was understood as aiming at unrestricted power over another person more or less mixed with destructiveness; masochism as aiming at dissolving oneself in an overwhelmingly strong power and participating in its strength and glory" (Fromm, 1941, p. 191). As a totalitarian leader, Hitler was able to provide millions of Germans with a means of escape by submitting to a larger power. The emotional appeal of Nazi ideology lay in "its spirit of blind obedience to a leader and of hatred against racial and political minorities, its craving for conquest and domination, its exaltation of the German people and the 'Nordic Race'" (1941, p. 182).

Sullivan recognized the immediate value of *Escape from Freedom* and arranged a series of eight separate reviews written by such well-known scholars as Ruth Benedict. The reviews were published in *Psychiatry* in 1942. As Helen Swick Perry has noted, "It was an impressive array, and it was bound to annoy Karl Menninger if no one else" (Perry, 1982, p. 388). In fact, another Freudian stalwart, Otto Fenichel, wrote a caustic review and Menninger would go on to write his own negative assessment in *The Nation*. Menninger sought to ostracize Fromm from mainstream psychoanalysis once and for all, writing that: "Erich Fromm was in Germany a distinguished sociologist. His book is written as if he considered himself a psychoanalyst" (Menninger, 1942, p. 317) In his haste to dismiss Fromm for his interdisciplinarity, however, Menninger overlooked a singularly important fact: *Escape from Freedom* was one of the only psychoanalytic texts at the time to address the reality of fascism, thus laying bare the failure of mainstream psychoanalysts to address the deep social and political crises of the day.[6] In the end, *Escape from Freedom* received near universal acclaim and it continues to be widely read today. Yet at the time, the book created a virtually unbridgeable rift with the Freudians.

Escape from Freedom was the result of detailed observation, psychological awareness and moral outrage. Above all, it was shaped by Fromm's first-hand familiarity with the rise of the Nazism and the immense threat it posed. The spectre of right-wing extremism was present throughout Fromm's adult life in Germany. The Nazis were initially a fringe right-wing paramilitary group, made up of disaffected and nationalistic World War I veterans. After the so-called Munich Beer Hall Putsch in 1923, which landed Hitler in prison, the Nazis changed their tactics and become involved in organized politics. They had little early success, and because the government of the Weimar Republic had already survived multiple challenges – the hyperinflation of 1923, an attempted left-wing take over and a failed right-wing coup – there was no reason to believe it would necessarily fail. But in 1929, with the onset of the financial crisis of the Great Depression and mass unemployment, the Nazi party began its rapid ascent and became a visible political presence. Pitched battles with the communists and the growth of a virulent anti-Semitism soon followed, portending an ominous future.

Within a relatively short period of time, more and more Germans lent their support to Hitler. In September 1930, the Nazi Party gained 18% of the vote and became the second largest party in Reichstag. In July 1932, they gained 37% and became the largest party. In January 1933, Hitler was appointed Chancellor, and in March of that year, the Nazi Party gained over 44% of the vote. Decrees creating a one-party state and cementing Hitler's position as dictator were quickly passed. In short order, the Nazis banned all other political parties, outlawed trade unions, imprisoned their political opponents in concentration camps and enacted their racial ideology. With their assumption of power, anti-Semitism, with which Fromm was very likely familiar as an orthodox Jew in Frankfurt, took on a menacingly new form.

Marxism and psychoanalysis were high on the Nazi's list of targets. The works of Marx and Freud were both included in the infamous book burnings that took place in the late 1930s. Marxists and members of left-wing political groups faced arrest and imprisonment.

The Nazis referred to psychoanalysis as a "Jewish science," prohibited psychoanalysts from practicing and closed their institutes. As a German Jewish psychoanalyst employed by the Marxist-oriented Institute for Social Research, Fromm knew that life under the Nazi regime would change dramatically and that he faced the possibility of harassment and imprisonment.

Racial Terror and Exile

Fromm's decision to leave Germany cannot have been easy and was influenced by the time he spent outside the country in the preceding years. In the summer of 1931, Fromm fell ill with tuberculosis and travelled to Davos, Switzerland, to recuperate. He stayed in Davos on and off for the next three years. In 1933, Fromm additionally spent several weeks visiting Chicago and New York at the invitation of Horney who emigrated in 1932. As a result, Fromm was able to observe the troubling changes in German politics from afar, and in May 1934, he fled from Switzerland to the United States.

Once in New York, Fromm confronted the challenges of the immigrant: integrating into a new culture, learning a new language and fitting into a new professional context. We know relatively little about his personal experience of immigration or what being a newly arrived émigré was like for him. Fromm sought to keep details of his personal life separate from his professional scholarship, and he never engaged in any kind of public self-analysis. Those who knew him have described Fromm as "intensely private" (Landis, 2009, p. 137) and as "always a private person" (Tauber, 2009, p. 131). It is safe to assume that Fromm was not unaffected by the personal and political upheavals. Nor is it clear that he would necessarily have chosen to leave the country, culture or language in which he grew up, were it not for the rise of the Nazis and the threat they posed.

In the years that followed, Fromm followed the events in Germany with growing alarm. The Nazi regime's aggression towards its neighbors was matched by the persecution of its own citizens. Anyone deemed undesirable was in peril: Jews, Sinti, Roma, gays and lesbians, the mentally ill and political opponents of all stripes. In 1935, the Nuremberg laws stripped Jews of their citizenship and basic rights. As perilous as life for Jews who remained in Germany had become, the Kristallnacht pogrom proved to be the turning point (see Frie, 2018). On the night of November 9 and into the morning of November 10, 1938, belligerent mobs destroyed nearly 300 synagogues and thousands of Jewish-owned professional properties and residences throughout Germany and Austria. The destruction was greatest in Berlin and Vienna, home to the largest Jewish communities. Approximately 100 were murdered, many committed suicide and the first mass incarceration of Jewish men in concentration camps was carried out. After Kristallnacht, all possibility of Jewish emigration from Germany came to abrupt end. The policy of mass deportation to ghettos and extermination camps further east was set in place in late 1941 and reached its height in the following year.

Accounts of Fromm's life at the time make little mention of his separation from family and friends.[7] In 1934, after arriving in New York, Fromm sponsored an affidavit for his estranged wife, Frieda Fromm-Reichmann, enabling her to leave later that year. But many of his family members together with friends and colleagues were unable to find safety in time. When Fromm emigrated, his mother, Rosa Fromm (née Krause), chose to stay behind in Germany, believing, or at least still hoping that the ascent of the Nazis was a momentary madness. Fromm's father had already died in late 1933, but not before he witnessed the Nazi rise to power. He was from a small family and his brother fled to the United States, while Fromm's cousin and life-long friend, Gertrud Hunziker-Fromm, had left earlier to study in Switzerland and settled there.

Fromm stayed in close contact with his mother as the circumstances in Germany worsened. After Kristallnacht, Rosa recognized the gravity of her situation and Fromm sought to secure her exit. He obtained a monetary loan to pay the high fee required by the Nazis for her to leave Germany and arranged for his mother to travel to England. Rosa spent the next 18 months in England along with many other refugees, so-called friendly enemy aliens. But arranging permission for her to enter the United States also proved to be very difficult. The American policy for admitting European Jews had become more stringent, influenced by the anti-Semitism during the course of the 1930s.

In November 1938, Fortune Magazine (Fortune Editors, 2015) published an opinion poll that asked Americans whether the United States should increase its immigration quotas or encourage political refugees – the largest number of them Jewish – to flee oppression in the fascist states of Europe. Fully two-thirds of the respondents agreed with the proposition that "we should try to keep them out." In January 1939, less than three months after Kristallnacht, two-thirds of respondents to Gallop's American Institute of Public Opinion said they would not take in 10,000 German Jewish refugee children (see Tharoor, 2015). In June 1939, a little more than six months after Kristallnacht, American authorities turned away the M.S. St. Louis, a ship filled with refugees from Nazi Germany. Its 900 Jewish passengers were forced to return to Europe, where a third of their number would be murdered in the Holocaust.

After Fromm paid another hefty fee to the US authorities, Rosa was finally able to join him in New York in 1941. Rosa lived until 1959 but other family members were not as fortunate. Rosa had four siblings and several cousins. She had grown up in Berlin, and most of the Krause family still lived there. Among her relatives, many members of the younger generation left for countries as far and wide as Bolivia, Brazil, Chili, Russia, the United States, England and Switzerland. Those who remained in Germany, because they were unable to pay the large fee or were simply too old or frail to make the journey, faced persecution and deportation. Rosa's brother Martin Krause and his wife, and Rosa's sister, Sophie Engländer and her husband were deported; none survived. A similar fate awaited Rosa's cousin, Gertrud Brandt, her husband and their youngest son, who were sent to the ghetto of Ostrow-Lubelski and then a concentration camp. Gertrud's three other children experienced persecution, imprisonment and murder. Rosa's cousin, Therese Zehetner, and her husband died in Frankfurt in 1940. Had they lived longer, they too would have been deported.

The Holocaust also engulfed other important people in Fromm's life such as Karl Landauer. He had been a close colleague and friend of Fromm and Fromm-Reichman and a co-founder of the Frankfurt Psychoanalytic Institute. In 1933, Landauer and his family fled for Sweden and then made their way to the Netherlands, where they believed they had found safety. Landauer worked as a training analyst as they tried to establish some semblance of normal life, but it was short lived. The German invasion of the Netherlands in May 1940 imperilled the lives of every Dutch Jew and Jewish refugee. In 1943,

Landauer and his family were arrested and a year later deported to the concentration camp of Bergen-Belsen. Landauer died there in January 1945.

It is hard to overlook this tragic dimension in Fromm's life when considering his work in the late 1930s and early 1940s.[8] The unpublished correspondence of Fromm's family members reveals that news was continually shared between South America, the United States and Europe. Fromm came to play a central role in this letter exchange because he was one of the few family members to have an established income at the time. Fromm helped his relatives in whatever way he could, but draconian emigration policies and the prohibitive cost of exit visas severely limited what he was able to do. Staying connected was essential and the value of the letters that reached those who remained in Germany was beyond measure. Letter writing was one of the few means available to sustain those in need and perhaps also a balm to assuage the powerlessness experienced by those, like Fromm, who escaped Germany but could do little more than look on. From the safety of New York, Fromm sent money, attempted to secure exist visas and wrote words of encouragement, all the while watching the steady escalation of the hateful Nazi ideology.

We can only imagine how Fromm managed daily life while being a witness to the terrible fate that befell his family members. There are few direct clues. Fromm had a correspondence with an F. Favez, an administrator at the Institute de Researches Sociales in Geneva, who was helping Fromm to arrange an exit visa for a cousin that was imprisoned in a concentration camp. In a letter addressed to Favez and dated April 25, 1940, Fromm gives us a sense of how the perilous events were closing in on him: "My life is always the same, working pretty much and trying not to be overwhelmed by what is going on in the world. If we were to speak over the phone now our conversations would not be so different from what they were then, excepting that things have become still worse."[9]

At the time, Fromm could not know how much worse the situation would become. Rainer Funk, who was Fromm's last personal assistant and the executor of his estate, has relayed to me that there was one letter amongst Fromm's belongings that he kept with him throughout his life. It was from his Aunt Sophie, written in Berlin on August 29th, 1942, on the eve of her deportation to Theresienstadt.

Sophie addressed the letter to her daughter in Chile, who then shared it with her cousin, Erich. The letter reads in part:

> We will probably go there [Theresienstadt] in the next while, but do not know the exact date yet. We are glad that we will see others there again. Father Breslauer's friend, Dr. Alexander, is there too. Likewise, Aunt Flora and countless friends and acquaintances. Aunt Hulda leaves her apartment the day after tomorrow. It is supposed to be good for us old people there, especially with the climate and the surroundings.
>
> Regrettably, regrettably, Martin and Johanna are not there [but in the Warsaw Ghetto.] We haven't heard from them in weeks and I am terribly worried as Uncle Martin was still weakened by his bile disease. Just stay healthy and don't worry about us. I always repeat it in every letter, because I do not know which one will reach you: we have had many good and beautiful things in life, wonderful children and grandchildren, in whom we have the greatest joy. That is worth so much; when you're old, you really know what that means.

At the end of the letter, the last Sophie would ever send, she asks her daughter to "send my dearest greetings to Tante Rosinchen [Erich Fromm's mother] and to Erich."[10] After leaving for Theresienstadt, Sophie and her husband were never heard from again.

Much of Fromm's energy during this period was directed towards developing *Escape from Freedom*. The book had a long gestation period and Fromm finished it only after Kristallnacht, as the fearsome persecution of Jews in Germany was compounded by a significant rise in anti-Semitism in the United States. Despite the dire circumstances, or perhaps precisely because of them, Fromm ends *Escape from Freedom* on a hopeful note. He suggests that democracy will be victorious over "the forces of nihilism" if it can imbue people with "the faith in life and in truth and in freedom" (1941, p. 238). Fromm was ultimately proven correct, but when he wrote those words, he could hardly know that the Second World War would rage on with unparalleled destructiveness until 1945. Nor could Fromm imagine that millions of Jewish lives would be extinguished in the Holocaust, including those of his own family members.

The traumatic effects of the Holocaust came in the form of letters from afar, but they were also present for Fromm in other ways (on the traumatic effects of the Holocaust and the legacy of German perpetration see Frie, 2017). In 1941, Fromm married Henny Gurland, a German-Jewish émigré from Frankfurt who had recently arrived in New York. Prior to 1933, Gurland had worked as a photographer for the newspaper of the Social Democratic Party in Germany. After fleeing for France, Gurland escaped the Gestapo a second time by undertaking a daring night time passage by foot over the Pyrenees into Spain (see Fittko, 2000). Gurland's companion on that harrowing journey was the German-Jewish writer and philosopher, Walter Benjamin. Gurland and her son survived the ordeal and eventually reached New York. But Benjamin tragically ended his own life after

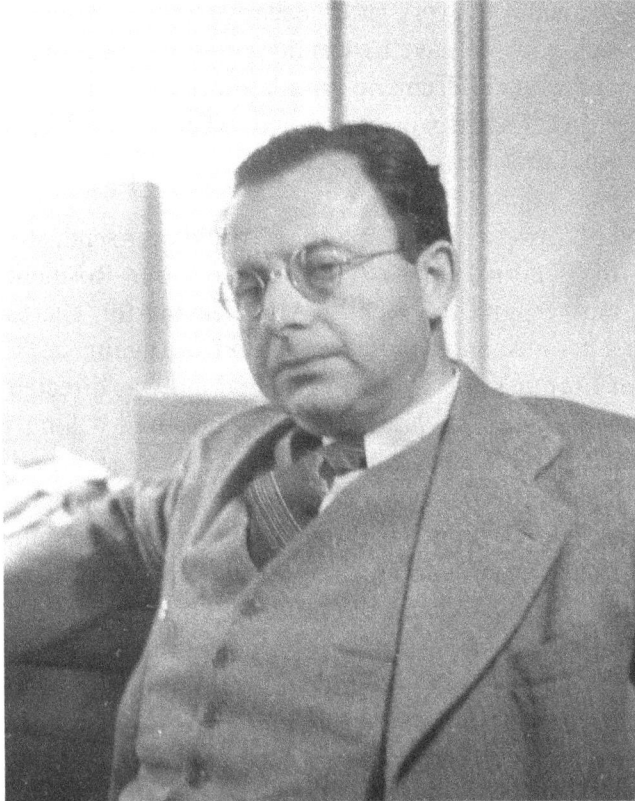

Figure 10 Erich Fromm in 1945, photo by Henny Gurland, ©Literary Estate of Erich Fromm, Tübingen.

being arrested by Spanish border guards in the town of Portbou. Benjamin had attempted an escape from France before and knew that he would be handed over to the Gestapo. Gurland was the last to speak with him before he died. Fromm met Gurland not long after, and the fact that they shared a common language, culture and understanding of the events in Europe undoubtedly drew them together. Despite their best efforts, Fromm and Gurland could do little to save family members, friends and colleagues they left behind. When the full scale of the catastrophe was revealed in the coming years, Fromm's faith in life was surely tested.

The Threat of Anti-Semitism

Escape from Freedom is notable for its account of the irrational appeal of authoritarianism, but there is little mention of the Nazi's hateful racial ideology. Nor does Fromm explain how anti-Semitism became such a powerful force in Germany. Instead, he focuses chiefly on lower middle-class support for Hitler.[11] Fromm's emphasis on socioeconomic class structure over ideology is in line with his Marxist orientation, and it would take historians and scholars alike some time before there was a concerted effort to explain and understand the role of anti-Semitism in Nazi Germany.

The absence of any discussion of anti-Semitism gives pause and leads to the question of whether and to what extent Fromm's lived experience may have shaped his approach. Since Fromm provides few personal details, any attempt to grapple with this question inevitably involves some measure of interpretation. What we do know is that Fromm was an émigré who was trying to adjust to a new cultural environment in which anti-Semitism was powerfully ascendant. Being identified as a recently-arrived German-Jewish intellectual who writes about anti-Semitism held certain risks. It meant potentially becoming a target of prejudice, which was a reason he did not remain in Germany. We can also wonder whether writing about anti-Semitism when he was actively involved in finding ways to save family members, friends and colleagues who were unable to leave Nazi Germany may have proven too painful.

Looking back, we find that it was Sullivan, not Fromm, who addressed the threat of anti-Semitism. Sullivan's detailed editorial on anti-Semitism and its effects was published in November 1938, in the second issue of *Psychiatry*. The fact that the editorial's publication coincided with the *Kristallnacht* pogrom can only have increased its impact on readers. Sullivan wrote about the escalation in anti-Jewish discrimination as well as the historical roots of anti-Semitism and the role played by Christianity in its propagation. In an important passage, Sullivan points to the dangers that anti-Semitism poses for all nations, and especially for functioning democracies:

> The most widespread hatred of a collectivity in the Western world today is antisemitism. Hatred of Jews has been made a national creed by at least one state. A trend in this direction is being manifested by the other totalitarian powers, and there is a disturbing responsiveness to the formula in many of the citizens of more democratic countries. Hatred under any circumstances can scarcely be constructive. It is essentially a destructive motivation.... Any pervasive enmity within democracy is dangerous. It increases the proportion of people who feel insecure. It intensifies feelings of individual differences. It undermines that general respect for other people which is the real basis for dependable self-respect. Antisemitism is this very sort of pervasive enmity. It is also an enmity peculiarly difficult to combat because of its particular irrational basis.
>
> (Sullivan, 1938, pp. 593–594)

What is unspoken in Sullivan's editorial is the personal understanding he brought to the subject. Sullivan's interactions with Sapir and Fromm (among others) would have made him directly aware of the realities of anti-Semitism and its pernicious effects. Sullivan had a close connection with Sapir and his family that stretched back to their first meeting in Chicago in 1926. For Sapir, anti-Semitism was an often-hostile aspect of the academic world he inhabited, especially at Yale University, which in the early 1930s employed very few Jewish faculty members and had a history of anti-Jewish discrimination (see Perry, 1982). And although Fromm did not write about his personal experience, Sullivan would in all likelihood have learned about the plight of his family members in Germany from their close interactions at the time.

We can also justifiably ask whether it was because Sullivan was not Jewish that he could more easily engage the subject of anti-Semitism than Fromm (or Sapir for that matter). To be sure, Sullivan struggled with societal prejudices in other ways. As a gay man, he was careful to hide his sexual orientation from public view given the high degree of public and private homophobia at the time. Thus, while Sullivan wrote articles on anti-Semitism and the effects of racism on young African-American men in the Deep South and the border states (Sullivan, [1940] 1964a and [1941] 1964b; see Wake and Stephens, this volume), he never wrote explicitly about homophobia. In a similar sense, Fromm engaged the twin spectres of authoritarianism and fascism but did not discuss the racist ideology that ensured his own exile and led to the murder of beloved family members and friends.

Racial Narcissism and White Supremacy, Past and Present

In the aftermath of World War II and the horrors of the Holocaust, the theme of human destructiveness held Fromm's attention. In 1964, at the height of the civil rights movement in the United States, Fromm published *The Heart of Man*, which builds on the arguments of *Escape from Freedom* and speaks more directly to the insidious nature of racism.[12] Fromm addresses the racial terror inflicted on African Americans and draws a direct link to the treatment of Jews in Nazi Germany.

During the 1950s and 1960s, the civil rights movement sought to end the segregation and disenfranchisement of African Americans. The movement met some of its fiercest opposition in the state of Alabama. In 1963, the white supremacist bombing of the 16th Street Baptist Church in Birmingham caused the death of 4 young African American girls. That same year, the state's Governor, George Wallace, declared in his inaugural address: "In the name of the greatest people that have ever trod this earth, I draw the line in the dust and toss the gauntlet before the feet of tyranny, and I say segregation now, segregation tomorrow, segregation forever." Fromm must have had Wallace's statement in mind when he wrote:

> The narcissistic conviction of the superiority of whites over blacks in parts of the United States and in South Africa demonstrates that there is no restraint to the sense of self-superiority or of the inferiority of another group. However, the satisfaction of a group requires also a certain degree of confirmation in reality. As long

as the whites in Alabama or in South Africa have the power to demonstrate their superiority over the blacks through social, economic, and political acts of discrimination, their narcissistic beliefs have some element of reality and thus bolster up the entire narcissistic thought-system. The same held true for the Nazis.

(Fromm, 1964, pp. 82–83)

Fromm is describing, in effect, how southern white supremacy enforced racial segregation through a system of Jim Crow laws at the state and local levels. Once in power in Germany, Hitler and the Nazi party enacted a series of similar laws that were directly based on their study of American race law. As the legal scholar James Whitman points out, it was not only "the Jim Crow South that attracted Nazi lawyers. In the early 1930s the Nazis drew on a rage of American examples, both federal and state. Their America was not just the South; it was a racist America write much larger" (Whitman, 2017, p. 5).

Our understanding of the direct connections that exist between Nazi Germany and the United States of the 1930s is relatively recent. Fromm would probably not have known that Nazi lawyers actually travelled to the United States to study American race law, but he knew enough from his experience of living in Germany to draw a direct connection between "racial narcissism which existed in Hitler's Germany, and which is found in the American South." In a manner reminiscent of *Escape from Freedom*, Fromm suggests that it was the social and economic anxieties experienced by many whites that created an especially fertile ground for their racism. "Economically and culturally deprived" whites who have no "realistic hope of changing" their situation; they have "only one satisfaction ... being superior to another racial group that is singled out as inferior." According to Fromm, members of this group feel that "'even though I am poor and uncultured I am somebody important because I belong to the most admirable group in the world – I am white;' or, 'I am Aryan'" (1964, p. 76). As Fromm adds, "If one examines the judgement of poor whites regarding blacks, or of the Nazis in regard to Jews, one can easily recognize the distorted character of their respective judgments ... the lack of objectivity often leads to disastrous circumstances" (1964, p. 81).

Turning to the nature of narcissism itself, Fromm suggests that racial narcissism of the group and the malignant narcissism of individuals is directly related. They are both "crudely solipsistic as well as xenophobic" (1964, p. 74). As Fromm explains, "the group narcissism of the 'whites' or the 'Aryans' is as malignant as the extreme narcissism of a single person can be" (1964, p. 77). The narcissism of the group and the individual are further connected by the way in which the group seeks a leader who can reflect and strengthen the group's narcissism.

> The highly narcissistic group is eager to have a leader with whom it can identify itself. The leader is then admired by the group which projects its narcissism onto him. In the very act of submission to the powerful leader, which is in depth an act of symbiosis and identification, the narcissism of the individual is transferred onto the leader. The great the leader, the greater the follower. Personalities who as individuals are particularly narcissistic are the most qualified to fulfill this function. The narcissism of the leader who is convinced of his greatness, and who has no doubts, is precisely what attracts the narcissism of those who submit to him. The half-insane leader is often the most successful one
>
> (Fromm, 1964, pp. 83–84)

When Fromm was writing *Escape from Freedom* in the late 1930s, he had already identified how the act of submitting to a powerful leader could assuage a group's anxieties. But Fromm could not know at that time just how dangerous and irrational the symbiotic relationship between the group and its leader could become. In *The Heart of Man*, he describes Hitler as "a man of extreme personal narcissism, who stimulated the group narcissism of millions of Germans" (1964, p. 82). He writes that fanatical leaders like Hitler needs "to find believers, to transform reality so that it fits their narcissism and to destroy all critics" (1964, p. 74). As Fromm puts it, "Here was an extremely narcissistic person who probably could have suffered a manifest psychosis had he not succeeded in making millions believe in his own self-image, [and] take his grandiose fantasies regarding the millennium of 'the Third Reich' seriously" (1964, p. 74).

Fromm's observations in *Escape from Freedom* and *The Heart of Man* not only help us to understand the sociopsychological dynamics of racism and xenophobia at the time (see also Fromm, 1973). His conclusions also have a powerful contemporary resonance and point us in the directly of a socially engaged psychoanalysis. The economic uncertainty and powerlessness of groups of workers in the face of neoliberal policies and globalism has given rise to leaders and movements eager to harness their anxiety and secure support for right-wing agendas. This process is reminiscent of the uncertainty that many Germans experienced in the aftermath of World War I and ultimately hastened the rise of Nazism in the 1930s. Historically distinct periods are difficult to compare, yet the upsurge in right-wing extremism, populism and racist and xenophobic agendas is common to each. Indeed, it is hard to read Fromm's analysis in *The Heart of Man* without thinking about the neo-Nazi rally in Charlottesville, Virginia, in 2017, or the way in which the actions of the far-right have often been implicitly, if not explicitly supported by populist leaders. The presidency of Donald Trump, for example, relied on nativism and race-baiting to secure support from its base of overwhelmingly white supporters, thus giving voice to the historically-entrenched racial divisions in American society. In her work, *Caste: The Origins of our Discontents*, Isabel Wilkerson (2020) suggests that Fromm's work on the pathology of racial narcissism not only helps to explain the racism of the past, it also evokes and sheds light on the underlying caste system that supports systemic racism and white supremacy in the United States today.

Fromm's life and work demonstrates that we are all inalterably shaped by social and political forces. The trauma and tragedy that engulfed his family during the Holocaust was an experience and a warning about human destructiveness that remained with Fromm through the remainder of his life. While Fromm became popularly known as a purveyor of hope and optimism, throughout his long career he returned again and again to the ways in which a socially and politically conscious psychoanalyst might respond to the dual threats of authoritarianism and racism. While psychoanalytic engagement with racism is often assumed to be a recent phenomenon, the work of Fromm (and Sullivan) suggests otherwise. The aim of this chapter has been to examine Fromm's contributions in their historical context and to consider the links between the past and present. In light of the social crises we fact today, I believe that Fromm, the psychoanalyst and the social critic, still has much to teach us. The pioneers of interpersonal psychoanalysis, like the historical contexts out of which their work emerged, deserve our attention.

Notes

1. See R. Funk (2001).
2. My account of Fromm's early life benefits from the work undertaken by three of Fromm's biographers: Burston, 1991; Funk, 2019; and Friedman, 2013.
3. Although Fromm descended from a long line of rabbis and had a devout Jewish upbringing, Fromm abandoned orthodox Judaism at the age of 26. In a 1962 interview, Fromm states: "I gave up my religious convictions and practices because I just didn't want to participate in any division of the human race, whether religious or political" (cited in Smith, 1980).
4. Today we would expand the influence of the patriarchal family constellation to also include such factors as the representations of gender in social media, gendered forms of language and performative social action, to name but a few.
5. Fromm's clinical perspective is often not well known or understood. For a collection of perspectives, in addition to some of Fromm's key clinical papers, see Funk, 2009.
6. Wilhelm Reich self-published the book, *The Mass Psychology of Fascism* in German in 1933, but it did not appear in English until 1946. In contrast to Fromm, who was concerned with the social forces that shape individuals and groups, Reich used a more traditional psychoanalytic lens to explain fascism as a consequence of sexual repression at the level of family and community.
7. I will return to the unpublished Fromm family correspondence below. Funk's unpublished German language essay (2005) is the only existing research I know of that directly addresses the letters of Fromm and his family members during the Holocaust. A general account of the family's tragic fate in the Holocaust can be found in Friedman (2013, pp. 70–76).
8. Our lack of knowledge about Fromm's decision to leave Germany is not unusual when we consider the general tenor of most postwar immigration narratives. In the decades after the Second World War, accounts of immigration by European Jewish émigrés and refugees were often framed in terms of freedom from oppression and the opportunity to prosper. The immediate postwar decades were defining period for Jewish refugee families. The overwhelming focus on cultural adaptation, perseverance and financial success shaped how many refugees talked about the past. Once in the United States, émigrés and refugees found themselves in a cultural milieu that was often uninterested in hearing about their experience. There was little room for talk of hardship, suffering or trauma. Adaptation to this new setting often meant focusing on the future while revealing little about the past (see Stein, 2014). It was not until the 1960s that Jewish communities and scholars began to employ the term "Holocaust," a process that was spurred in part by the

publication of Raul Hillberg's pathbreaking book *The Destruction of the European Jews* in 1961. And it was not until the airing of the television mini-series of the same name "Holocaust" in 1978 that the term entered into general usage in the American public (see Lipstadt, 2016).

9. Quoted with permission from Rainer Funk, Director of the Erich Fromm Archive in Tübingen, Germany, where the letters are housed.

10. This excerpt is published by permission of Rainer Funk, Director of the Fromm Archive in Tübingen, Germany. The translation is my own and it forms part of a longer, forthcoming study I am completing of the Fromm family Holocaust letters and the place of this history in Fromm's life and work. See also Funk, 2019, pp. 91–92.

11. Fromm believed that the German lower middle classes were Hitler's primary source of support. The focus on social-economic class reflected his Marxist orientation. However, as it turned out, the Nazis appealed to members of all social-economic classes and support for Hitler was present to varying degrees throughout Germany.

12. See also Fromm's important work from 1973, *Anatomy of Human Destructiveness*, which is beyond the scope of this chapter and which I take up in my aforementioned and forthcoming extended study.

References

Adorno, T., Frenkel-Brunswik, E., Levinson, D. and Sanford, N. (1950). *The authoritarian personality*. New York: Harper and Brothers.

Burston, D. (1991). *The legacy of Erich Fromm*. Cambridge, MA: Harvard University Press.

Fittko, L. (2000). *Escape through the Pyrenees*. Evanston, IL: Northwestern University Press.

Fortune Editors (Nov. 18, 2015). Here's Fortune's Survey on How Americans Viewed Jewish Refugees in 1938. *Fortune Magazine*. Retrieved from: https://fortune.com/2015/11/18/fortune-survey-jewish-refugees/

Frie, R. (2014). Cultural psychoanalysis: Psychoanalytic anthropology and the interpersonal tradition. *Contemporary Psychoanalysis*, 50, 371–394.

Frie, R. (2017). *Not in My Family: German Memory and Responsibility after the Holocaust*. New York: Oxford University Press.

Frie, R. (Ed.) (2018). *History flows through us: Germany, the Holocaust and the importance of empathy*. New York: Routledge.

Friedman, L. J. (2013). *The lives of Erich Fromm: Love's prophet*. New York: Columbia University Press.

Fromm, E. (1930). Psychoanalysis and sociology. In Bronner, S.E. and Kellner, D. (Eds.), *Critical theory and society: A reader* (pp. 37–39). London: Routledge, 1989.

Fromm, E. (1934). The theory of mother right and its relevance for social psychology. In *The crisis of psychoanalysis: Essays on Freud, Marx, and social psychology* (pp. 84–109). New York: Holt, Rinehart and Winston, 1970.

Fromm, E. (1937). Man's impulse structure and its relation to culture. In Funk, R. (Ed.), *Beyond Freud: From individual to social psychology* (pp. 17–74). New York: American Mental Health Foundation, 2010.

Fromm, E. (1939). The social philosophy of "will therapy." *Psychiatry*, 2, 229–237.

Fromm, E. (1941). *Escape from freedom*. New York: Farrar & Rinehart.

Fromm, E. (1949). Psychoanalytic characterology and its application to the understanding of culture. In Sargent, S.S. and Smith, M. W. (Eds.), *Culture and personality* (pp. 1–12). New York: Viking Press.

Fromm, E. (1964). *The heart of man: Its genius for good and evil*. Riverdale, NY: American Mental Health Foundation Books, 2010.

Fromm, E. (1973). *The anatomy of human destructiveness*. New York: Holt, Rinehart and Winston.

Fromm. E. (1984). *The working class in Weimar Germany: A psychological and sociological study*. Cambridge, MA: Harvard University Press.

Funk, R. (2001). Erich Fromm's role in the foundation of the IFPS: Evidence from the Erich Fromm Archives in Tübingen. *International Forum of Psychoanalysis*, 9, 187–197.

Funk, R. (2005). *Erleben von Ohnmacht im Dritten Reich: Das Schicksal der jüdischen Verwandtschaft Erich Fromms aufgezeigt an Dokumenten*. Unpublished manuscript. Fromm Archive, Tübingen.

Funk, R. (Ed.) (2009). *The clinical Erich Fromm: Personal accounts and papers on therapeutic technique*. New York: Rodopi Press.

Funk, R. (2019). *Life itself is an art: The life and work of Erich Fromm*. New York: Bloomsbury Academic.

Horney, K. (1939). Can you take a stand? In Paris, B. J. (Ed.), *The unknown Karen Horney: Essays on gender, culture and psychoanalysis* (pp. 222–227). New Haven, CT: Yale University Press, 2000.

Landis, B. (2009). When you hear the word, the reality is lost. In Funk, R. (Ed.), *The clinical Erich Fromm: Personal accounts and papers on therapeutic technique* (pp. 137–140). New York: Rodopi Press.

Lipstadt, D. (2016). *Holocaust: An American understanding*. Rutgers, NJ: Rutgers University Press.

McLaughlin, N. (1999). Origin myths in the social sciences: Fromm, the Frankfurt School and the emergence of critical theory. *Canadian Journal of Sociology*, 24, 109–139.

McLaughlin, N. (2017). Who killed off Fromm's reputation in North America? Russell Jacoby's *Social Amnesia* and the forgetting of a public intellectual. *Fromm Forum*, 21, 7–21.

Menninger, K. (March 14, 1942). Loneliness in the Modern World. *The Nation*, 154.

Perry, H. S. (1982). *Psychiatrist of America: The life of Harry Stack Sullivan*. Cambridge, MA: Harvard University Press.

Smith, J. Y. (1980, March 19). Psychoanalyst and philosopher Erich Fromm dies. *The Washington Post*. Retrieved from: https://www.washingtonpost.com

Stein, A. (2014). *Reluctant witnesses: Survivors, their children and the rise of Holocaust consciousness*. New York: Oxford University Press.

Sullivan, H. S. (1938). Antisemitism. *Psychiatry*, 1, 593–598.

Sullivan, H. S. (1940). Discussion of the case of Warren Wall. In *The fusion of psychiatry and social science* (pp. 100–107). New York, NY: Norton, 1964a.

Sullivan, H. S. (1941). Memorandum on a psychiatric renaissance. In *The fusion of psychiatry and social science* (pp. 89–95). New York, NY: Norton, 1964b.

Tauber, E. (2009). Words are ways. In Funk, R. (Ed.), *The clinical Erich Fromm: Personal accounts and papers on therapeutic technique* (pp. 131–134). New York: Rodopi Press.

Tharoor, I. (Nov. 17, 2015). What Americans thought of Jewish Refugees on the eve of World War II. *The Washington Post*. Retrieved from: https://www.washingtonpost.com

Thompson, C. (1956). Sullivan and Fromm. *Contemporary Psychoanalysis*, 15, 195–200, 1979.

Wake, N. (2011). *Private practices: Harry Stack Sullivan, the science of homosexuality, and American liberalism*. New Brunswick, NJ: Rutgers University Press.

Whitman, J. Q. (2017). *Hitler's American model: The United States and the making of Nazi race law*. Princeton, NJ: Princeton University Press.

Wilkerson, I. (2020). *Caste: The origin of our discontents*. New York: Random House.

Index